Anesthesia for Patients Too Sick for Anesthesia

Guest Editors

BENJAMIN A. KOHL, MD
STANLEY H. ROSENBAUM, MD

ANESTHESIOLOGY CLINICS

www.anesthesiology.theclinics.com

Consulting Editor
LEE A. FLEISHER, MD, FACC

March 2010 • Volume 28 • Number 1

SAUNDERS an imprint of ELSEVIER, Inc.

W.B. SAUNDERS COMPANY
A Division of Elsevier Inc.

1600 John F. Kennedy Boulevard, Suite 1800 • Philadelphia, PA 19103-2899

http://www.theclinics.com

ANESTHESIOLOGY CLINICS Volume 28, Number 1
March 2010 ISSN 1932-2275, ISBN-13: 978-1-4377-1795-2

Editor: Rachel Glover
Developmental Editor: Donald Mumford

Anesthesiology Clinics (ISSN 1932-2275) is published quarterly by Elsevier Inc., 360 Park Avenue South, New York, NY 10010-1710. Months of issue are March, June, September, and December. Periodicals postage paid at New York, NY and at additional mailing offices. Subscription prices are $134.00 per year (US student/resident), $268.00 per year (US individuals), $328.00 per year (Canadian individuals), $417.00 per year (US institutions), $517.00 per year (Canadian institutions), $189.00 per year (Canadian and foreign student/resident), $372.00 per year (foreign individuals), and $517.00 per year (foreign institutions). To receive student and resident rate, orders must be accompanied by name of affiliated institution, date of term, and the *signature* of program/residency coordinator on institutions letterhead. Orders will be billed at individual rate until proof of status is received. Foreign air speed delivery is included in all *Clinics'* subscription prices. All prices are subject to change without notice. POSTMASTER: Send address changes to *Anesthesiology Clinics,* Elsevier Health Sciences Division, Subscription Customer Service, 3251 Riverport Lane, Maryland Heights, MO 63043. Customer Service (orders, claims, online, change of address): Elsevier Health Sciences Division, Subscription Customer Service, 3251 Riverport Lane, Maryland Heights, MO 63043. Tel:1-800-654-2452 (U.S. and Canada); 314-447-8871 (outside U.S. and Canada). Fax: 314-447-8029. E-mail: journalscustomerservice-usa@elsevier.com (for print support); journalsonlinesupport-usa@elsevier.com (for online support).

Reprints. For copies of 100 or more of articles in this publication, please contact the Commercial Reprints Department, Elsevier Inc., 360 Park Avenue South, New York, NY 10010-1710. Tel.: 212-633-3812; Fax: 212-462-1935; E-mail: reprints@elsevier.com.

Anesthesiology Clinics, is also published in Spanish by McGraw-Hill Inter-americana Editores S. A., P.O. Box 5-237, 06500 Mexico D. F., Mexico.

Anesthesiology *Clinics,* is covered in *MEDLINE/PubMed (Index Medicus), Current Contents/Clinical Medicine, Excerpta Medica, ISI/BIOMED,* and *Chemical Abstracts.*

Printed and bound by CPI Group (UK) Ltd, Croydon, CR0 4YY

Transferred to Digital Print 2011

Contributors

CONSULTING EDITOR

LEE A. FLEISHER, MD, FACC
Robert D. Dripps Professor and Chair of Anesthesiology and Critical Care, University of Pennsylvania School of Medicine, Philadelphia, Pennsylvania

GUEST EDITORS

BENJAMIN A. KOHL, MD
Assistant Professor of Anesthesiology and Critical Care; Director, Critical Care Fellowship, University of Pennsylvania School of Medicine, Philadelphia, Pennsylvania

STANLEY H. ROSENBAUM, MD
Professor of Anesthesiology, Internal Medicine and Surgery; Vice-Chair, Department of Anesthesiology, Yale University School of Medicine, New Haven, Connecticut

AUTHORS

ROSS BLANK, MD
Clinical Lecturer, Division of Critical Care Medicine, Department of Anesthesiology, University of Michigan Medical Center, University of Michigan Medical School, Ann Arbor, Michigan

JAMES M. BLUM, MD
Clinical Lecturer, Division of Critical Care Medicine, Department of Anesthesiology, University of Michigan Medical Center, University of Michigan Medical School, Ann Arbor, Michigan

TRICIA E. BRENTJENS, MD
Associate Clinical Professor, Member, Division of Critical Care, Department of Anesthesiology, Columbia University; Medical Director, Post Anesthesia Care Unit, New York Presbyterian Hospital, Presbyterian Campus, New York, New York

GERALDINE DAUMERIE, MD
Fellow, Cardiac Anesthesia, Department of Anesthesiology, Hospital of the University of Pennsylvania, Philadelphia, Pennsylvania

JONATHAN FROGEL, MD
Attending Staff Anesthesiologist, Department of Anesthesiology, Henry Ford Hospital, Detroit, Michigan

DRAGOS GALUSCA, MD
Chief Resident, Department of Anesthesiology, Henry Ford Hospital, Detroit, Michigan

EMILY K.B. GORDON, MD
Department of Anesthesiology and Critical Care, University of Pennsylvania School
of Medicine, Philadelphia, Pennsylvania

ALA S. HADDADIN, MD, FCCP
Assistant Professor, Division of Cardiothoracic Anesthesia and Adult Critical Care Medicine; Medical Director Cardiothoracic Intensive Care Unit, Department of Anesthesiology, Yale University School of Medicine, New Haven, Connecticut

GARY E. HILL, MD, FCCM
Professor, Department of Anesthesiology and Pain Management, The University of Texas Southwestern Medical Center, Dallas, Texas

JENNIFER E. HOFER, MD
Resident Physician, Department of Anesthesia and Critical Care, The University of Chicago Hospitals, Chicago, Illinois

BENJAMIN A. KOHL, MD
Assistant Professor of Anesthesiology and Critical Care; Director, Critical Care Fellowship, University of Pennsylvania School of Medicine, Philadelphia, Pennsylvania

CHANHUNG Z. LEE, MD, PhD
Assistant Professor, Department of Anesthesia and Perioperative Care, University of California, San Francisco, San Francisco, California

LAWRENCE LITT, MD, PhD
Professor, Department of Anesthesia and Perioperative Care, University of California, San Francisco, San Francisco, California

ANNA V. LOGVINOVA, MD
Senior Resident, Department of Anesthesia and Perioperative Care, University of California, San Francisco, San Francisco, California

MAUREEN MCCUNN, MD, MIPP, FCCM
Assistant Professor, Department of Anesthesiology and Critical Care, University of Pennsylvania School of Medicine, Philadelphia, Pennsylvania

DAWOOD NASIR, MD
Assistant Professor, Department of Anesthesiology and Pain Management, The University of Texas Southwestern Medical Center, Dallas, Texas

MARK E. NUNNALLY, MD
Associate Professor, Department of Anesthesia and Critical Care, The University of Chicago Hospitals, Chicago, Illinois

E. ANDREW OCHROCH, MD, MSCE
Associate Professor, Department of Anesthesiology, Hospital of the University of Pennsylvania; Department of Surgery, Division of Thoracic Surgery, University of Pennsylvania, Philadelphia, Pennsylvania

CHRISTOPHER J. O'CONNOR, MD
Professor, Department of Anesthesiology, Rush University Medical Center, Chicago, Illinois

BABATUNDE OGUNNAIKE, MD
Associate Professor, Department of Anesthesiology and Pain Management,
The University of Texas Southwestern Medical Center, Dallas, Texas

LAURYN R. ROCHLEN, MD
Clinical Lecturer, Division of Critical Care Medicine, Department of Anesthesiology,
University of Michigan Medical Center, University of Michigan Medical School,
Ann Arbor, Michigan

ROBERT B. SCHONBERGER, MD, MA
Fellow in Cardiothoracic Anesthesia, Department of Anesthesiology, Yale University
School of Medicine, New Haven, Connecticut

STANLEY SCHWARTZ, MD
Clinical Associate Professor, Director, Diabetes Disease Management, Department
of Medicine, Philadelphia Heart Institute, University of Pennsylvania Health System,
Philadelphia, Pennsylvania

THOMAS H. SCOTT, MD
Department of Anesthesiology and Critical Care, University of Pennsylvania School
of Medicine, Philadelphia, Pennsylvania

STACEY SU, MD
Assistant Professor, Department of Surgery, Division of Thoracic Surgery, University
of Pennsylvania, Philadelphia, Pennsylvania

KENNETH J. TUMAN, MD
The Anthony D. Ivankovich Professor and Chair, Department of Anesthesiology, Rush
University Medical Center, Chicago, Illinois

GEBHARD WAGENER, MD
Assistant Professor, Chief, Division of Vascular Anesthesia; Member, Division of Critical
Care, Department of Anesthesiology, Columbia University, New York, New York

WILLIAM L. YOUNG, MD
Professor and Vice Chair, Department of Anesthesia and Perioperative Care, University
of California, San Francisco, San Francisco, California

Contents

This review outlines the perioperative anesthesia considerations of patients with vascular diseases of the central nervous system, including occlusive cerebrovascular diseases with ischemic risks and various cerebrovascular malformations with hemorrhagic potential. The discussion emphasizes perioperative management strategies to prevent complications and minimize their effects if they occur. Planning the anesthetic and perioperative management is predicated on understanding the goals of the therapeutic intervention and anticipating potential problems.

The acutely septic patient is a multifaceted challenge for the anesthetist. Unlike most elective surgery patients, acutely septic patients have severe systemic disease before the physiologic insults of anesthesia and surgery. The decision to operate is usually informed by the urgent or emergent need to correct a severe surgical problem and weighed against the higher risks of morbidity and mortality from the procedure itself. The care of the septic patient in the intensive care unit can help guide operating room management. However, the acuity and time course of intraoperative events, including hemorrhage and drug-induced shock states, compel the anesthetist to respond aggressively with therapies that may or may not be strongly substantiated with long-term data in the intensive care unit setting. The anesthesiologist must place considerations concerning short-term survival from the acute insult of surgery ahead of longer-term considerations.

The critically ill patient who requires anesthesia is frequently a concern for the anesthesiologist. In addition to having potential hemodynamic lability and coagulopathy, the critically ill patient frequently experiences profound respiratory failure. The approach to the patient requiring advanced ventilatory support requires an understanding of respiratory failure, the pathophysiology causing respiratory failure and hypoxia, the physiology of mechanical ventilation and the advanced modes of ventilation available in the intensive care unit (ICU). This article discusses the basic definitions of hypoxia and common pathologic states, reviews the physiology of mechanical ventilation and advanced forms of ventilation available in the ICU, and concludes with recommendations for the management of patients with severe respiratory failure when they are taken to the operating room.

Anesthesiologists often care for patients with renal insufficiency or renal failure. These patients may present to the operating room for a minor procedure such as an inguinal hernia repair or an arteriovenous fistula/graft. Alternatively, they may present for major abdominal operations or coronary artery bypass grafting. Critically ill patients presenting to the operating room may have acute kidney injury. It is imperative that the anesthesiologist understands the ramifications of renal failure and adjusts the anesthetic plan accordingly. Hemodynamic monitoring and fluid management can be challenging in this patient population. Various metabolic abnormalities can ensue that the anesthesiologist must be able to manage in the acute setting of the operating room.

This article reviews the current state of knowledge of the pathophysiology, diagnosis, and treatment of acute coronary syndrome outside and during the perioperative period. It highlights some aspects of relevance for the anesthesiologist caring for these patients. Perioperative modalities for the management of patients suffering from this syndrome, the major guidelines and the evidence behind them, and possible avenues for future research is explored.

Patients with valvular heart disease represent a growing segment of the population and can present major challenges to clinical anesthesiologists. This review focuses on patients with advanced left-sided valvular disease undergoing noncardiac surgery. The pathophysiology and anesthetic implications of aortic stenosis and insufficiency and mitral stenosis and insufficiency are discussed, with a focus on optimizing perioperative management and decision making for patients with these conditions.

The anesthetic management of patients with pericardial tamponade is challenging, as they present with not only the cardiovascular compromise that defines pericardial tamponade, but often have comorbid conditions that increase the complexity of their management. This review describes the pathophysiology, etiology, clinical presentation, and anesthetic management of patients with pericardial tamponade, with an emphasis on the intraoperative period and the management of pericardial window procedures, the most common clinical scenario where anesthesiologists will encounter pericardial tamponade.

Trauma is the third leading cause of death in the U.S. Timely acute care anesthetic management of patients following traumatic injury may improve outcome. Recognition of highly-mortal injuries to the brain, heart, lungs, liver, and pelvis should guide trauma-specific management strategies. Rapid intraoperative treatment of life-threatening conditions following injury includes the use of 'controlled-under resuscitation' of fluid administration until surgical hemorrhage control, early factor replacement in addition to transfusion of packed red blood cells, and use of adjuvant therapies such as recombinant factor VIIa. These treatment strategies, other recent developments in acute trauma resuscitation, and a review of associated co-existing medical conditions that may impact mortality, are presented.

Organ toxicity caused by poisons or drug therapy is diverse and may not be commonly encountered clinically. In general, commonly encountered conditions caused by drug/toxin pharmacology can be classified into 7 categories by shared mechanisms of organ injury. This review of drug/toxin-induced injury discusses drug or toxin-induced pathology that the clinician may encounter and therapeutic approaches to these syndromes.

Patients with endocrinopathies frequently present to the operating room. Although many of these disorders are managed on a chronic basis, patients may have acute changes in the perioperative period that, if left unrecognized, can have a negative effect on perioperative morbidity and mortality. It is imperative that anesthesiologists understand the implications of the surgical stress response on hormonal flux. This article focuses on the 4 most commonly encountered endocrinopathies: diabetes mellitus, hyperthyroidism, hypothyroidism, and adrenal insufficiency. Specific challenges pertaining to patients with pheochromocytoma are also discussed.

Tracheal stenosis may occur secondary to trauma, tumors, infection, inflammatory diseases, or iatrogenic causes. Understanding these lesions requires a basic understanding of the physics of airflow. All of these patients must be carefully evaluated and require a series of tests, including pulmonary function tests and radiographic studies. Treatment of tracheal lesions is a multidisciplinary issue and requires the close participation of interventional pulmonologists, anesthesiologists, and surgeons.

THE CLINICS ARE NOW AVAILABLE ONLINE!

Access your subscription at:
www.theclinics.com

Foreword

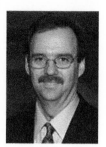

Lee A. Fleisher, MD
Consulting Editor

With the constant advances in anesthesiology, patients with increasing comorbidities are being brought to the operating room by our surgical colleagues. Patients who were once too sick for anesthesia are now routinely cared for with good outcomes. Yet, our goal must be to get these patients through the surgery without a further deterioration in organ dysfunction. In this issue of the *Anesthesiology Clinics*, an outstanding group of contributors have provided us with insights into how best care for these patients.

As Guest Editors for this issue, we are fortunate to have Benjamin A. Kohl, MD and Stanley H. Rosenbaum, MD. They both have the unique background of training in internal medicine, anesthesiology, cardiac anesthesia, and critical care. Ben is Assistant Professor of Anesthesiology and Critical Care at the University of Pennsylvania and Director of the Fellowship in Critical Care. He has extensive clinical research experience related to perioperative glucose management. Stan is Professor of Anesthesiology, Medicine and Surgery at Yale University School of Medicine where he is Vice Chair for Academic Affairs and Director of the Section of Perioperative and Adult Anesthesia. He is currently focusing his interests on medical ethics. Together they have developed an outstanding issue.

Lee A. Fleisher, MD
University of Pennsylvania School of Medicine
3400 Spruce Street, Dulles 680
Philadelphia, PA 19104, USA

E-mail address:
Lee.fleisher@uphs.upenn.edu

doi:10.1016/j.anclin.2010.02.001
1932-2275/10/$ – see front matter © 2010 Elsevier Inc. All rights reserved.

Preface
Anesthesia for Patients Too Sick for Anesthesia

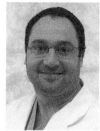   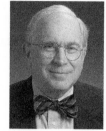

Benjamin A. Kohl, MD   Stanley H. Rosenbaum, MD
Guest Editors

By their very nature, surgical patients are "sick"—some more so than others. Anesthesiologists, however, are accustomed to creating a very low-risk environment for their patients. Hence, in the setting of *severe disease*, the anesthesiologist has a very powerful tendency to want to view such a patient as "too sick for anesthesia." We believe that this viewpoint, while long-standing and deeply ingrained in traditional anesthesiology practice, is in conflict with a modern view of aggressive surgical care. Severe surgical disease necessitating urgent or emergency surgery often coexists with severe medical illnesses.

If anesthesiologists canceled every patient who presented with multiple comorbidities, our operating rooms would be empty. Indeed, it is because of our unique training and skill-set that we are in a position to care for these critically ill patients. The balance between underlying medical problems and the need to provide surgical therapy must include careful consideration of the risks and benefits. However, only with a comprehensive understanding of the underlying pathology and its effect on anesthesia can a decision be made to proceed with the surgery despite significant medical dangers. Hence we have created this volume entitled (only partially facetiously), "Anesthesia for patients [traditionally regarded as] too sick for anesthesia."

We and our authors have focused on a group of common, but potentially severe, medical conditions in the environment of surgical disease in an effort to provide a guide and resource for the anesthesiologist to become more familiar with these medical problems.

Anesthesiology Clin 28 (2010) xv–xvi
doi:10.1016/j.anclin.2010.01.012
1932-2275/10/$ – see front matter © 2010 Elsevier Inc. All rights reserved.

anesthesiology.theclinics.com

We are grateful to Lee. A. Fleisher, MD, the series editor for *Anesthesiology Clinics of North America*, for his guidance and advice. We are also thankful for the support of Rachel Glover and the publishing team at Elsevier.

Benjamin A. Kohl, MD
Department of Anesthesiology and Critical Care
University of Pennsylvania School of Medicine
3400 Spruce Street, Dulles 680
Philadelphia, PA 19104, USA

Stanley H. Rosenbaum, MD
Department of Anesthesiology
Yale University School of Medicine
Yale-New Haven Hospital
789 Howard Avenue
PO Box 208051
New Haven, CT 06520, USA

E-mail addresses:
Benjamin.Kohl@uphs.upenn.edu (B.A. Kohl)
stanley.rosenbaum@yale.edu (S.H. Rosenbaum)

Anesthetic Concerns in Patients with Known Cerebrovascular Insufficiency

Anna V. Logvinova, MD, Lawrence Litt, MD, PhD,
William L. Young, MD, Chanhung Z. Lee, MD, PhD*

KEYWORDS

• Anesthesia • Cerebrovascular disease • Cerebral ischemia
• Brain vascular malformation • Intracranial hemorrhage

Insufficient blood flow to all or part of the brain, or *cerebrovascular insufficiency*, can be caused by *cerebrovascular diseases*, whereby one or more blood vessels that supply brain tissue have structural and functional abnormalities that cause permanent or episodic brain ischemia or hemorrhage. Cerebrovascular diseases can often be characterized as either *occlusive* (eg, carotid and intracranial arterial stenosis), or *hemorrhagic*, with this term applying to vascular disorders whose natural course proceeds to hemorrhage, as with various cerebrovascular malformations (eg, intracranial aneurysms and arteriovenous malformations). Cerebrovascular diseases have remained a third leading cause of death in the United States, with an estimated 500,000 new cerebrovascular accidents (CVAs) each year.[1] Cerebrovascular diseases are the most disabling of all neurologic disorders, causing a residual neurologic deficit in more than 50% of survivors, and necessitating chronic care for more than 25% of survivors.[1]

Advances in acute CVA management have steadily increased survival at different stages of recovery. For intracranial cerebrovascular malformations, as a result of the trend in favor of more conservative medical management,[2,3] there will be an increase in the group of patients at risk for hemorrhagic stroke. Thus the population of patients who need to be anesthetized for nonneurologic surgeries and interventions includes an increasing number with cerebrovascular diseases, causing additional, unique, anesthesia-related challenges and concerns. Prevention strategies to avoid cerebral ischemia or hemorrhage must be embedded in plans for anesthesia management at all stages of perioperative care. The preoperative assessment should include an evaluation of the patient's cerebrovascular status as a potential source of perioperative

Department of Anesthesia and Perioperative Care, University of California, San Francisco, 1001 Potrero Avenue, Room 3C-38, San Francisco, CA 94110, USA
* Corresponding author.
E-mail address: CLee4@anesthesia.ucsf.edu

Anesthesiology Clin 28 (2010) 1–12
doi:10.1016/j.anclin.2010.01.007   anesthesiology.theclinics.com

morbidity and mortality. A comprehensive review is needed of concurrent pathologies, comorbidities, and medications that might influence the perioperative course. Defining cerebrovascular reserve and ischemic and hemorrhagic risks in the type of surgery that is planned must be tailored to each patient's particular lesions. Plans and preparations need to be made in advance of interventions that might be needed to deal with complications or emergencies. Anesthetic planning should be especially clear about hemodynamic goals and monitoring. This article presents detailed anesthetic concerns for the most common cerebrovascular diseases.

ANESTHETIC CONCERNS FOR OCCLUSIVE CEREBROVASCULAR DISEASES
Carotid and Vertebral Arteries

Carotid arteries provide approximately 80% of cerebral blood flow (CBF) while vertebral arteries supply the remaining 20%. Between 5% and 10% of people older than 65 years were found to have carotid stenosis of more than 50%.[4,5] The etiology of occlusive diseases is complex, and includes genetic and environmental factors. Major risk factors of occlusive diseases are atherosclerosis, embolic events, and hypertension. Common carotid occlusions, followed by vertebrobasilar occlusions, are typically found in the older patient population. Adequate cerebral circulation in patients with occlusive disease is normally maintained by 2 mechanisms: *cerebral autoregulation*, which allows sustained CBF across a wide range of perfusion pressures, also known as "cerebral reserve," and *collateral blood flow* from the circle of Willis and other pathways.[6] Stenotic lesions decrease or exhaust cerebral reserve. In the case of cerebrovascular stenosis, the brain area supplied distal to the stenotic portion can become hypoperfused when the cerebral perfusion pressure decreases to below the passive-pressure range on the autoregulation curve. Additional collateral blood supply through the ophthalmic artery or through the external carotid arteries, mainly involving facial circulation, may have developed in particular cases.[6,7]

Anesthetic management of patients with occlusive cerebrovascular diseases is challenging because of the high morbidity and dynamic nature of these diseases, and coexisting pathologies specific or nonspecific to ischemic stroke. Protection from further cerebral ischemia, by supporting adequate cerebral perfusion pressure (CPP) to maintain CBF in potential ischemic regions in patients with known cerebrovascular stenosis, is a key consideration for anesthesiologists during perioperative periods.

Preoperative Preparation

Preoperative assessment should be approached with the goal of preventing new or repeated episodes of cerebral ischemia. Timing, symptoms, extent, and etiology of any previous ischemic events should be carefully noted. If the ischemic episode occurred in the previous 4 weeks, the conventional approach is that all elective surgery should be postponed. However, post-stroke changes in central nervous system physiology, such as impaired cerebral autoregulation, increased permeability of the blood-brain barrier, and loss of CO_2 responsiveness, can persist for more than 4 weeks.[8–11] All acute and residual neurologic deficits should be assessed and documented if new neurologic deficits occur postoperatively.

A diagnostic workup, if it has not been done, should be pursued to find the cause. The workup should include Doppler studies of carotid and vertebrobasilar arteries and brain magnetic resonance angiography (MRA). Such studies can be important in discussions with neurologists and surgeons about the risks and benefits of definitive revascularization procedures of occlusive lesions before conducting a nonneurologic elective surgical procedure. Moreover, such studies can help guide the management of perioperative care by providing a better understanding of the underlying pathology. Diffusion-weighted magnetic resonance imaging (MRI) is often useful in evaluating for silent ischemic lesions in patients with recent transient ischemic attacks (TIAs) without obvious neurologic deficits, particularly when a cardiovascular or other major procedure is planned. However, little is known about correlations between silent ischemic lesions and postoperative neurologic complications.[12,13] Nonetheless, all available original and follow-up brain imaging study results should be reviewed.

As before all anesthesia cases, the airway, head, and neck should be examined to identify airway problems or evidence of positional ischemia. Anesthetic agents, especially in the presence of long-term antihypertensive therapy, may lead to a CBF decrease that exacerbates ischemia in the areas perfused distal to fixed stenotic lesions. Decisions on use of antihypertensive therapy versus blood pressure augmentation should be based on baseline blood pressure, clinical status of the patient, and regimen of thrombolytic therapy, because there is a higher risk for cerebral edema and hemorrhage in the presence of hypertension. Noting neurologic deficits, contractures, and neuralgias is also very important when planning for regional or neuroaxial anesthesia, because potential exacerbation of preexisting neurologic deficits may develop after regional anesthesia.[14,15]

Coexisting disease workups should include major organ system reviews, considering that there is a large percentage of serious comorbidities in this patient population. Cardiovascular history and examination are very important, with emphasis on preoperative baseline blood pressure for each patient. Cardiac workup should include, at minimum, a baseline electrocardiogram (ECG) to document arrhythmias and ST abnormalities. Transthoracic echocardiography (TTE) may be employed to assess global cardiac function, valvular and wall-motion abnormalities, and intracardiac thrombi. Transesophageal echocardiography (TEE) could be especially helpful to thoroughly evaluate the aorta and left atrial appendage for sources of emboli.

Pulmonary problems, including aspiration and nosocomial pneumonia, and both central and obstructive sleep apnea, are commonly seen. A baseline chest radiograph should be obtained. A sleep study should be considered if sleep apnea is suspected.

Patients can also have dysphagia, gastroesophageal reflux disease (GERD), and gastropathy.[16] Nutritional status should be assessed; in chronically malnourished intensive care unit (ICU) patients, uninterrupted total parenteral nutrition should be considered intraoperatively.

The fluid and electrolyte status of these patients should be analyzed with a full set of laboratory tests. Common electrolyte disturbances could be pathogenic or iatrogenic (caused by mannitol administration and fluid resuscitation in the acute phase, and antihypertensive diuretics in the chronic phase). Chronic and acute renal insufficiency may be present. Radiographic contrast can augment renal insufficiency. It is often useful to learn from the radiologist if a patient's serum creatinine should be expected to have a contrast-induced increase from a particular diagnostic study. Hemodialysis-dependent patients present an additional challenge because of their cardiovascular and electrolyte instability; patients should be dialyzed before surgery.

Diabetes mellitus is commonly found in these patients. Hyperglycemia has been suggested as an independent poor outcome predictor in patients with focal cerebral ischemia.[17] Lactic acidosis occurs during ischemic episodes due to anaerobic metabolism in a setting of systemic hypoperfusion; it potentially could increase neuronal cell death if prolonged cerebral ischemia is also produced. Normoglycemia should be maintained by managing perioperative stress, avoiding glucose-containing solutions, and using volume expansion and insulin, which also has a glucose-independent effect on brain protection. Hypoglycemia can be more detrimental to the injured brain than hyperglycemia. The NICE SUGAR trial showed that the tight goal of blood glucose levels of 80 to 100 is associated with up to 5% of episodes of hypoglycemia in ICU patients, and with increases in mortality as well.[18] Blood glucose levels of 100 to 180 are deemed safer in ICU patients; however, it has yet to be studied in CVA patients in a perioperative setting. Blood glucose should be closely monitored and titrated with an insulin protocol for diabetic patients.

Hematology studies should be obtained, including complete blood count and coagulation studies, because anticoagulation and antiplatelet therapy can be part of prevention strategies in patients with known high risk for stroke. The decision needs to be made whether to continue, bridge, or stop anticoagulants and antiplatelet agents depending on the patient's thrombosis risks, as well as plans for neuroaxial and regional interventions.

Chronic care patients in nursing homes and other settings may present with specific issues such as skin breakdown, multidrug-resistant flora, bone fractures in various stages of healing due to falls, cognitive decline, and depression.

Intraoperative Management

In brief, cerebral protection, in the form of support of CPP, prevention of reduced CBF, and further embolization, is the main goal of every stage of anesthesia. When deciding on intravenous agents like midazolam or fentanyl for preinduction or sedation, there is a fine line between the patient's comfort and the ability to maintain adequate ventilation and oxygenation. Detrimental effects, including worsening of neurologic status, delirium, or even the reappearance of a prior focal neurologic deficit that has been transient and thought to be repaired, may occur.[19,20] It has been demonstrated that small doses of either midazolam or fentanyl can induce transient focal motor deterioration in patients with prior motor deficits.[20] With more sophisticated methodology, it has also been shown that not only motor functions but also language and spatial functions can be affected.[21] These observations have been extended to include neurologically intact patients with a recent history of TIA, who had negative diffusion-weighted imaging but still suffered from a reemergence of prior focal deficits after intravenous midazolam administration.[21] Despite these risks, opiates and benzodiazepines are safe when used with caution.

In cases of general anesthesia, intraoperative monitoring and adequate intravenous access decisions should be tailored to the type of surgical procedure, especially if large fluid shifts, associated hemodynamic instability, hypotension, and reduction in oxygen-carrying capacity and delivery are anticipated. Standard American Society of Anesthesiologists monitors—continuous ECG monitoring with ST-segment trends, ventilation monitoring, and continuous temperature monitoring—should be applied to every patient. Beat-to-beat arterial pressure monitoring and blood sampling can be facilitated by arterial line. Preinduction monitoring of invasive arterial blood pressure should be established and correlated to noninvasive cuff pressures in patients with high cerebral ischemic potential. Blood pressure support and stability within a reasonable range of "normotensive" for each particular patient is of utmost importance for maintaining adequate CPP and protecting the brain from further ischemia.[22] Induction of general anesthesia should be performed with extra caution, considering coexisting airway problems, aspiration potential due to lack of protective reflexes, dysphagia, and gastric dysmotility, as well as high likelihood of obstructive sleep apnea. The choice of anesthetic agent should take into account rapid and smooth emergence to facilitate postoperative neurologic assessment as soon as possible. Inhalational or total intravenous techniques or combinations of these have been successfully employed. There is no clear superiority of one modern inhaled anesthetic over another in terms of pharmacologic protection against neuronal damage. Depolarizing neuromuscular blockade should be generally avoided beyond 1 week post stroke or if the duration is unknown. Upper motor neuron lesions and prolonged immobilization may cause upregulation of skeletal muscle acetylcholine receptors, with a resulting risk of hyperkalemia on administration of depolarizing neuromuscular relaxants (succinylcholine). Relative normocapnia should be maintained unless intracranial pressure (ICP) is a concern.[23] Arterial blood gas, electrolytes, and glucose should be monitored throughout surgery, depending on the status and type of procedure, and abnormalities should be corrected as needed. Maintaining hematocrit at around 30% may help to ensure optimal oxygen delivery to areas at ischemic risk.[24,25] Emergence and extubation must be approached as carefully as intubation, because the same risks for upper airway obstruction, aspiration, and difficult airway still apply. Blood pressure surges should be avoided with careful titration of antihypertensives. Patients should be extubated when they become fully awake.

Postoperative Care

Postoperatively, the neurologic status of these patients should be assessed as soon as possible. Delirium and worsening preexisting or reappearing deficits need to be documented and closely followed. Pain should be monitored and managed well, as it represents one of the direct sympathetic stimulants leading to catecholamine release and extreme postoperative hypertension, which may increase incidence of ischemia. Tight cardiovascular control should be continued with all appropriate monitors including continuous beat-to-beat arterial pressure. Early postoperative recovery of respiratory function may be challenging in patients with known sleep apnea, dysphagia, aspiration problems, and pulmonary abnormalities. Positive pressure noninvasive ventilation like continuous positive airway pressure or Bi-Pap should be used only if patients can cooperate, and if there are no contraindications like altered mental states and problems with airway protection.

Moyamoya Disease

Moyamoya disease is a rare occlusive cerebrovascular disease[26,27] that manifests as cerebral ischemia (with more common presentation in children) or cerebral hemorrhage (with more common initial presentation in adults). In addition to presenting for commonly seen surgical interventions, patients with this debilitating progressive disease often present for ongoing angiography follow-ups, and neurosurgical revascularization procedures.

This disease is characterized by angiographic findings of progressive intracranial carotid artery stenosis, and development of a fine network of collateral vessels at the brain base. These vessel clusters are termed *moyamoya* ("puff of smoke" in Japanese), and diagnosed by cerebral angiography. Intracranial aneurysms can be associated with Moyamoya disease.[14,28] There is also an association with neurofibromatosis, tuberous sclerosis, neuromuscular dysplasia, and subsequent traumatic insult. Moyamoya is considered to be a systemic disease, with typical pathologic features in the affected arteries, including renal artery stenosis, and abdominal and coronary arteries stenosis.[29] Treatment is focused on prevention of ischemia, and consists of surgical creation of direct or indirect anastomosis of the superficial temporal artery to the middle cerebral artery or various indirect extra-to-intracranial bypasses. Mainstay medical therapy includes vasodilators and combinations of antiaggregants and anticoagulants. Prognosis is usually poor, with significant neurologic morbidity.

Perioperative Concerns

Preexisting neurologic deficits and history of ischemia and hemorrhages should be documented in preoperative assessment. Angiographic findings should be studied, including the presence of concurrent cerebral aneurysms. Collegial decisions regarding ongoing anticoagulation need to be made together with the surgery team; if possible anticoagulants should be discontinued, to prevent excessive intraoperative bleeding.

Management of anesthesia involves dealing not only with cerebral ischemia prophylaxis but also with problems that pediatric patients are typically predisposed to, for example, frequent upper respiratory infections, laryngospasm, strong vagal reflexes, and fluid-dependent cardiac output. The goals of anesthesia include hemodynamic stability, because hypotension could cause regional cerebral ischemia and severe hypertension may lead to hemorrhage. If at all possible, an arterial line should be placed prior to induction of anesthesia for beat-to-beat arterial blood pressure monitoring. Sevoflurane inhalational induction is a frequent route for children. Any intravenous induction agents can be used safely, perhaps with the exception of ketamine. Hemodynamic instability during intubation and other stimulating points should be blunted by narcotics, esmolol, or propofol. Volatile anesthetics and intravenous agents have been successfully used for anesthesia maintenance. It has been reported that propofol anesthesia can potentially provide cerebral protection and preserve regional CBF in frontal lobes, and is associated with lower ICP compared with sevoflurane anesthesia.[30] These findings warrant further investigation.

The patients' vasoreactivity to hypocapnia is slightly reduced, but not generally compromised.[31] Tagawa and colleagues[32] determined that there is a regional decrease in CBF as the mean value of $PaCO_2$ decreases from 39 to 29. Therefore, any activity resulting in hyperventilation and hypocapnia in children, for example, crying, is dangerous and can be associated with TIAs.[33] Children are apt to become excited and cry during the perioperative period; therefore, excitement should be addressed with premedication and a clear postoperative plan for pain and emesis management.

Hypovolemia should be treated with colloid or normotonic crystalloid if there is any concern regarding cerebral edema. Anemia should be treated to avoid additional cerebral ischemia. A smooth and rapid emergence facilitates postoperative neurologic examination as soon as possible, because postoperative complications may include new ischemic stroke, hemorrhage, or seizures/postictal states.

ANESTHETIC CONCERNS FOR HEMORRHAGIC CEREBROVASCULAR DISEASE
Cerebral Aneurysms

Intracranial aneurysms have a prevalence of between 1% and 5% in the adult population,[2] and 20% to 50% of all aneurysms may rupture in a person's lifetime depending on the risk factors. Aneurysmal subarachnoid hemorrhage, contributing to 5% to15% of stroke cases, has a 30-day mortality rate of 45% with many survivors suffering substantial long-term disability. Development of cerebral aneurysms is likely to be multifactorial, most cases being sporadic. A small portion of them may belong to dissecting aneurysms formed as a result of arterial wall trauma, mycotic aneurysms caused by infection and often associated with subacute bacterial endocarditis, and pseudoaneurysms as a result of abrupt severe arterial trauma. Sometimes they can be associated with conditions like Marfan syndrome, Ehler-Danlos syndrome, adult polycystic renal disease, and fibromuscular dysplasia.[34]

With the increased availability of and improvement in technology, many intracranial aneurysms are asymptomatic incidental findings during autopsy or routine imaging studies. Certain risk factors for rupture have been identified, and preventive treatment in the form of endovascular or open aneurysm clipping has been recommended for high-risk lesions.[35] A systematic review of existing studies brought together 24 different risk factors associated with higher risk of subarachnoid hemorrhage.[36] The history of subarachnoid hemorrhage, large size, and posterior circulation location were all identified as independent predictors for aneurysm rupture. Other risk factors include female gender (1:4 male to female ratio, especially after the age of 50), advanced age, nonwhite ethnicity, hypertension, low body mass index, smoking, and alcohol consumption.

Prevention of rupture and hemorrhage in patients harboring intracranial aneurysms during the perioperative period requires meticulous coordination of hemodynamic and ventilation management. One key consideration here is the proper management of transmural pressure, which serves as an indication of aneurysm wall tension, defined as the difference between mean arterial pressure (MAP) and ICP. An emerging concept suggests that another key component of the pathophysiology of intracranial aneurysms is sustained abnormal vascular remodeling coupled with inflammation and increase of proinflammatory cytokine production. Surgery and perioperative period are associated with increased inflammatory reactions, which may exacerbate the pre-existing inflammatory state thus creating a particularly "favorable" environment for aneurysm rupture. Identifying these potential targets may provide a new treatment strategy that would aim to stabilize the aneurysms by reducing inflammation and vascular remodeling for the perioperative period.[33,37]

Preoperative Preparation

Aneurysm rupture is a catastrophic event in the perioperative period. Reliable information regarding the risks of cerebral aneurysm rupture is needed to help formulate an anesthetic preventive plan. Risk factors for aneurysmal rupture should be carefully assessed preoperatively in patients with unruptured cerebral aneurysms. Duration after the diagnosis of disease needs to be considered, as aneurysms may grow in size or change morphology and hemodynamics. These changes, along with worsening comorbidities including proinflammatory states, may convert aneurysms from fairly innocent to highly dangerous.

Thorough evaluation of coexisting diseases, including cardiovascular and pulmonary status, should be performed, with emphasis on preoperative blood pressure history and hypertension management. The patient's antihypertensive therapy should be optimized if possible.

Intraoperative Management

The anesthesia plan should be formulated considering hemorrhagic potential of the lesion(s), keeping in mind that the risk of bleeding is always present regardless of how "low risk" an aneurysm seems to appear. Hemodynamic goals should be set to allow for maintenance of adequate CPP while simultaneously minimizing aneurysm transmural pressure, ideally around a preoperative "normotensive" level determined for each patient. Excessive hyperventilation may decrease ICP and, as a consequence, increase transmural pressure across the aneurysm, which can potentially lead to rupture of the aneurysm. Because a similar concern regarding transmural pressure holds for the surgeon's intraoperative opening of the dura, the anesthesiologist should be particularly attentive at that time during the case.

Hemodynamic stability should be pursued with a high priority during induction and intubation, although modest fluctuation in blood pressure within 20% of baseline levels may be permitted. There is a presumed risk for rupturing an aneurysm with severe arterial hypertension; however, there are no data to directly support this risk other than older case series reporting rupture during anesthetic induction in the range of about 1%, presumably as a result of acute hypertension. Therefore, the actual risk may be much lower with currently improved monitoring and anesthetic techniques. Nevertheless, the conventional wisdom is to maintain the systolic blood pressure at 20% to 30% of baseline levels.

Postoperative Care

Hypertension after emergence from general anesthesia is common in this patient population, especially in those with a history of chronic hypertension. In the case of an increase of more than 20% of baseline above the patient's preoperative levels, the blood pressure needs to be controlled by using β-blockers or other antihypertensive medications. Neurologic examinations should be performed as early as possible to rule out any gross neurologic deficits that could be a sign of possible intracranial events.

Arteriovenous Malformations

Brain arteriovenous malformations (AVM) represent a relatively rare but significant cause of severe neurologic morbidity and mortality of associated hemorrhage in younger adults. Brain AVMs have a prevalence of 10 to 18 per 100,000 adults,[38] and a new detection rate of approximately 1.3 per 100,000 person-years.[39] The morphologic definition of AVM is a vascular mass (nidus), which is a complex tangle of abnormal vessels directly shunting blood between arterial and venous circulations without a capillary bed. Usually there is high flow through feeding arteries, nidus, and draining veins. Symptoms include intracranial bleeds, as well as chronic headaches, mass effects, and seizures. Spontaneous hemorrhage has been estimated to range approximately from 2% to 4% per year.[40] Hemorrhagic AVM presentation, increasing age, deep brain location, and exclusive deep venous drainage appear to be independent predictors for AVM hemorrhage during natural history follow-up. The risk of spontaneous hemorrhage may be as low as 0.9% in AVMs without these risk factors, but as high as 34.4% for those harboring all 3 risk factors.[41] Up to 10% of AVMs are associated with cerebral aneurysms that typically occur along feeding arteries that lead to AVMs due to high flow and pressure in these vessels, or within the nidus of the AVM itself.

Treatment modalities include surgical resection, embolization, and stereotactic therapy. The pathogenesis of AVMs has not been clearly established. At the molecular level, abnormal expression of angiogenesis and inflammatory proteins have been implicated, and nucleotide polymorphisms have been associated with AVM susceptibility and rupture, which may offer potential targets for medical therapy development.[42]

Perioperative Management

Perioperative anesthetic concerns in patients with known unruptured AVMs are similar to those with aneurysms; however, these patients are generally younger and could present with less systemic comorbidities. Hemodynamic stability is a primary goal for anesthetic management. Although an AVM rupture incidence due to blood pressure surges on induction is extremely rare, the general recommendation is to keep it as close as possible to the patient's baseline levels to avoid mitigating circumstances.[43] Despite intracranial pressure control being rarely a problem in AVM patients without hemorrhage, avoiding cerebral vasodilators and hypercarbia are reasonable considerations because decreased intracranial compliance may be present.

Equally important is a smooth and rapid emergence from general anesthesia, which is essential for facilitating immediate postoperative neurologic examinations to rule out adverse cerebrovascular events.

MANAGEMENT OF POTENTIAL PERIOPERATIVE NEUROLOGIC CRISES

Despite careful planning and management, perioperative neurovascular catastrophes can occur in patients with known cerebrovascular diseases. Recognizing characteristics of potential cerebrovascular events is the first key element in initiating interventions in response to emergencies. In the anesthetized patient, the sudden onset of bradycardia and hypertension (Cushing response) may be the only clue to a developing hemorrhage with acute intracranial pressure increase.[23] Both acute ischemic episodes and small vascular ruptures can be subclinical in patients under general anesthesia, and can manifest in the recovery period by failure to wake up, altered mental status, and possible focal neurologic deficits. In semi-awake patients undergoing procedures under monitored anesthesia care, acute occlusive lesions will be more clinically obvious. Bleeding catastrophes are usually heralded by headache, nausea, vomiting, and vascular pain related to the area close to the rupture. Sudden loss of consciousness is not always caused by intracranial hemorrhage. Seizures, as a result of transient ischemia and the subsequent postictal state, can also lead to an obtunded patient.

A clear resuscitation plan, coupled with rapid and effective communication between the anesthesia and surgery teams, is critical for good outcomes. The primary responsibility of the anesthesia team is to preserve gas exchange and, if indicated, secure the airway. For occlusive problems, the goal is to increase distal perfusion with or without direct thrombolysis; deliberate hypertension, titrated to neurologic examination and physiologic imaging studies, is recommended. For acute intracranial hemorrhage, blood pressure should be maintained at low normal levels; anticoagulation, if used, should be immediately reversed. Further resuscitation of intracranial bleed with increasing ICP includes bringing the head up to 15° in neutral position if possible, achieving normocapnia, or $PaCO_2$ manipulation consistent with clinical setting. Mannitol, 0.5 ~ 1.5 g/kg, can be given by intravenous infusion. The patient should be allowed to passively cool to low normal temperature, or be aggressively cooled if febrile. A ventriculostomy catheter can be considered for monitoring and treatment of increasing ICP. Patients with suspected thromboembolic events or rupture will require emergency computed tomography scan, but emergency craniotomy is usually not indicated. The aforementioned are generic recommendations. All drug doses must be adapted to clinical situations and in accordance with the patient's preexisting medical condition.

SUMMARY

Preoperative assessment, in addition to a completely documented neurologic examination and cerebrovascular risk prediction, should focus on the patient's cardiac, pulmonary, renal, and endocrine status. To prevent perioperative complications in patients with cerebrovascular diseases, anesthetic plans should emphasize understanding of the underlying pathophysiology, determining hemodynamic goals, and anticipating potential perioperative crisis while being prepared to intervene.

REFERENCES

1. National Center for Health Statistics. Health, United States, 2007, with chartbook on trends in the health of Americans 2007. Available at: http://www.ncbi.nlm.nih. gov/books/bv.fcgi?indexed=google&rid=healthus07.chapter.trend-tables. Accessed November 1, 2009.
2. Wiebers DO, Whisnant JP, Huston J 3rd, et al. Unruptured intracranial aneurysms: natural history, clinical outcome, and risks of surgical and endovascular treatment. Lancet 2003;362(9378):103–10.
3. The ARUBA Trial. A randomized trial of unruptured brain arteriovenous malformations 2009. Available at: http://www.arubastudy.org/. Accessed December 8, 2009.
4. O'Leary DH, Polak JF, Kronmal RA, et al. Distribution and correlates of sonographically detected carotid artery disease in the Cardiovascular Health Study. The CHS Collaborative Research Group. Stroke 1992;23(12):1752–60.
5. Fine-Edelstein JS, Wolf PA, O'Leary DH, et al. Precursors of extracranial carotid atherosclerosis in the Framingham Study. Neurology 1994;44(6):1046–50.
6. Joshi S, Ornstein E, Young WL. Cerebral and spinal cord blood flow. In: Cottrell JE, Smith DS, editors. Anesthesia and neurosurgery. 4th edition. St Louis: Mosby; 2001. p. 19–68.
7. Gelabert HA, Moore WS. Occlusive cerebrovascular disease: medical and surgical considerations. In: Cottrell JE, Smith DS, editors. Anesthesia and neurosurgery. 4th edition. St Louis: Mosby; 2001. p. 459–72.
8. Meyer JS, Shimazu K, Fukuuchi Y, et al. Impaired neurogenic cerebrovascular control and dysautoregulation after stroke. Stroke 1973;4(2):169–86.
9. Finnigan SP, Walsh M, Rose SE, et al. Quantitative EEG indices of sub-acute ischaemic stroke correlate with clinical outcomes. Clin Neurophysiol 2007;118(11): 2525–32.
10. Takano T, Nagatsuka K, Ohnishi Y, et al. Vascular response to carbon dioxide in areas with and without diaschisis in patients with small, deep hemispheric infarction. Stroke 1988;19(7):840–5.
11. Zhao P, Alsop DC, Abduljalil A, et al. Vasoreactivity and peri-infarct hyperintensities in stroke. Neurology 2009;72(7):643–9.
12. Nagura J, Suzuki K, Johnston SC, et al. Diffusion-weighted MRI in evaluation of transient ischemic attack. J Stroke Cerebrovasc Dis 2003;12(3):137–42.
13. Latchaw RE, Alberts MJ, Lev MH, et al. Recommendations for imaging of acute ischemic stroke: a scientific statement from the American Heart Association. Stroke 2009;40(11):3646–78.
14. Vercauteren M, Heytens L. Anaesthetic considerations for patients with a pre-existing neurological deficit: are neuraxial techniques safe? Acta Anaesthesiol Scand 2007;51(7):831–8.
15. Veering BT. Regional anesthesia and the patient with preexisting neurological disease. Curr Opin Anaesthesiol 2009;22(5):634–6.
16. Schaller BJ, Graf R, Jacobs AH. Pathophysiological changes of the gastrointestinal tract in ischemic stroke. Am J Gastroenterol 2006;101(7):1655–65.
17. Weir CJ, Murray GD, Dyker AG, et al. Is hyperglycaemia an independent predictor of poor outcome after acute stroke? Results of a long-term follow-up study. BMJ 1997;314:1303–6.
18. Van den Berghe G, Bouillon R, Mesotten D. Glucose control in critically ill patients. N Engl J Med 2009;361(1):89 [author reply: 91–2].

19. Chollet F, DiPiero V, Wise RJ, et al. The functional anatomy of motor recovery after stroke in humans: a study with positron emission tomography. Ann Neurol 1991; 29(1):63–71.
20. Thal GD, Szabo MD, Lopez-Bresnahan M, et al. Exacerbation or unmasking of focal neurologic deficits by sedatives. Anesthesiology 1996;85(1):21–5.
21. Lazar RM, Fitzsimmons BF, Marshall RS, et al. Midazolam challenge reinduces neurological deficits after transient ischemic attack. Stroke 2003;34(3): 794–6.
22. Jellish WS. Anesthetic issues and perioperative blood pressure management in patients who have cerebrovascular diseases undergoing surgical procedures. Neurol Clin 2006;24(4):647–59, viii.
23. Young WL. Anesthesia for endovascular neurosurgery and interventional neuroradiology. Anesthesiol Clin 2007;25(3):391–412, vii.
24. Duebener LF, Sakamoto T, Hatsuoka S, et al. Effects of hematocrit on cerebral microcirculation and tissue oxygenation during deep hypothermic bypass. Circulation 2001;104(12 Suppl 1):I260–4.
25. Hare GM, Tsui AK, McLaren AT, et al. Anemia and cerebral outcomes: many questions, fewer answers. Anesth Analg 2008;107(4):1356–70.
26. Genetic and Rare Diseases Information Center (GARD). Moyamoya disease. Available at: http://rarediseases.info.nih.gov/GARD/Disease.aspx?PageID=4&26 DiseaseID=7064/Print. Accessed December 8, 2009.
27. Uchino K, Johnston SC, Becker KJ, et al. Moyamoya disease in Washington State and California. Neurology 2005;65(6):956–8.
28. Kawaguchi S, Sakaki T, Morimoto T, et al. Characteristics of intracranial aneurysms associated with moyamoya disease. A review of 111 cases. Acta Neurochir (Wien) 1996;138(11):1287–94.
29. Togao O, Mihara F, Yoshiura T, et al. Prevalence of stenoocclusive lesions in the renal and abdominal arteries in Moyamoya disease. AJR Am J Roentgenol 2004; 183(1):119–22.
30. Kikuta K, Takagi Y, Nozaki K, et al. Effects of intravenous anesthesia with propofol on regional cortical blood flow and intracranial pressure in surgery for Moyamoya disease. Surg Neurol 2007;68(4):421–4.
31. Karasawa J, Touho H, Kawaguchi M. Moyamoya disease: diagnosis and treatment. Neurosurg Q 1996;6(2):137–50.
32. Tagawa T, Naritomi H, Mimaki T, et al. Regional cerebral blood flow, clinical manifestations, and age in children with Moyamoya disease. Stroke 1987;18(5): 906–10.
33. Hashimoto T, Meng H, Young WL. Intracranial aneurysms: links between inflammation, hemodynamics and vascular remodeling. Neurol Res 2006;28(4):372–80.
34. Brisman JL, Song JK, Newell DW. Cerebral aneurysms. N Engl J Med 2006; 355(9):928–39.
35. Ishibashi T, Murayama Y, Urashima M, et al. Unruptured intracranial aneurysms: incidence of rupture and risk factors. Stroke 2009;40(1):313–6.
36. Clarke M. Systematic review of reviews of risk factors for intracranial aneurysms. Neuroradiology 2008;50(8):653–64.
37. Jayaraman T, Paget A, Shin YS, et al. TNF-alpha-mediated inflammation in cerebral aneurysms: a potential link to growth and rupture. Vasc Health Risk Manag 2008;4(4):805–17.
38. Arteriovenous Malformation Study Group. Arteriovenous malformations of the brain in adults. N Engl J Med 1999;340(23):1812–8.

39. Stapf C, Mast H, Sciacca RR, et al. The New York Islands AVM Study: design, study progress, and initial results. Stroke 2003;34(5):e29–33.
40. Kim H, Sidney S, McCulloch CE, et al. Racial/ethnic differences in longitudinal risk of intracranial hemorrhage in brain arteriovenous malformation patients. Stroke 2007;38(9):2430–7.
41. Stapf C, Mast H, Sciacca RR, et al. Predictors of hemorrhage in patients with untreated brain arteriovenous malformation. Neurology 2006;66(9):1350–5.
42. Kim H, Marchuk DA, Pawlikowska L, et al. Genetic considerations relevant to intracranial hemorrhage and brain arteriovenous malformations. Acta Neurochir Suppl 2008;105:199–206.
43. Ogilvy CS, Stieg PE, Awad I, et al. Recommendations for the management of intracranial arteriovenous malformations: a statement for healthcare professionals from a special writing group of the Stroke Council, American Stroke Association. Circulation 2001;103(21):2644–57.

Taking the Septic Patient to the Operating Room

Jennifer E. Hofer, MD*, Mark E. Nunnally, MD

KEYWORDS

• Sepsis • Critical illness • Anesthesia management

The acutely septic patient is a multifaceted challenge for the anesthetist. Unlike most elective surgery patients, they have severe systemic disease before the physiologic insults of anesthesia and surgery. Most septic patients will have had major organ dysfunction even before the onset of their acute illness. Consequently, this is a high-risk population. The decision to operate is usually informed by the urgent or emergent need to correct a severe surgical problem and weighed against the higher risks of morbidity and mortality from the procedure itself.

The care of the septic patient in the intensive care unit (ICU) can help guide operating room management. Modern critical care supports failing organs, prevents failures in others, and allows the process of healing to continue. Similar principles of care can benefit the septic patient who happens to be undergoing anesthesia and surgery. However, the acuity and time course of intraoperative events, including hemorrhage and drug-induced shock, compel the anesthetist to respond aggressively with therapies that may or may not be strongly substantiated with long-term data in the ICU setting. The anesthesiologist must make short-term survival from the acute insult of surgery the top priority.

Sepsis is the systemic manifestation of the body's response to infection. This is a particular version of the stress response. It affects virtually every organ system and therefore has many implications for the anesthesiologist. Anesthesiologists have unique skills at resuscitation, monitoring, and titration that make them well prepared to handle this therapeutic challenge.

HEMODYNAMIC EFFECTS

Sepsis can be characterized by extreme hemodynamic derangements, culminating in septic shock. This shock is hyperdynamic. Cardiac output typically increases and

---

This work was not funded and the authors do not have any financial connections to the work being published.

Department of Anesthesia and Critical Care, The University of Chicago Hospitals, 5841 South Maryland Avenue, MC 4028, Chicago, IL 60637, USA

* Corresponding author.

E-mail address: jhofer@dacc.uchicago.edu

Anesthesiology Clin 28 (2010) 13–24

doi:10.1016/j.anclin.2010.01.005   anesthesiology.theclinics.com blood flow is redistributed away from high-flow tissue beds. Systemic vascular resistance decreases. Venous capacitance with venous pooling reduces cardiac preload. Vascular permeability increases, causing more third-space fluid loss. In late sepsis, cardiac contractility can decrease. Elevated lactate levels may reflect tissue oxygen deficiency or altered metabolism.[1]

The anesthesiologist's goal in correcting these hemodynamic abnormalities should simply be to improve tissue perfusion. Adequate perfusion can be hard to measure and end points for resuscitation remain unclear. According to one theory, supranormal oxygen levels are called for to correct systemic oxygen debt. However, this theory has not been well supported. A more prudent course to improve outcomes is to provide a modest addition of volume or of vasoactive agents to maintain tissue perfusion pressure, titrated to patient response.[1]

Certain hemodynamic goals have been suggested. One literature-based practice is to maintain a central venous pressure (CVP) of 8 to 12 mm Hg, a mean arterial pressure greater than 65 mm Hg, urine output of at least 0.5 mL/kg/h, a hematocrit of greater than 30%, and a central venous oxygen saturation of greater than 70%.[2] These are, at best, rough guidelines. Each patient has different resuscitation requirements. Ultimately, organ perfusion indices inform decisions about the adequacy of resuscitation and circulatory support.

INDUCTION OF ANESTHESIA

Measures required to induce the septic patient are different from those for other patients because of altered pharmacokinetics and pharmacodynamics,[3] increased risk of cardiovascular toxicity, and enhanced patient sensitivity to sedative effects. Increases in the volume of drug distribution, resulting from expanded extracellular fluids, are common. Albumin levels are low and alpha-1 acid glycoprotein is elevated, changing the active free fraction of various anesthetic agents for their target receptors.

Patients with unstable hemodynamics, whether because of hypovolemia, cardiac dysfunction, impaired vasoregulation, or adrenal insufficiency from depleted vasopressin and cortisol, are highly sensitive to induction agents. Induction doses should be titrated to effect since full intubating doses may cause irreversible cardiovascular collapse. The choice of induction agent should be informed by its favorable and unfavorable properties.

The selection of etomidate for intubation of the septic patient may be the ultimate Faustian bargain because of the potential for adrenal suppression. This may be particularly relevant in sepsis, where adrenal insufficiency and its consequences are more common than in previously healthy patients. Etomidate is considered for intubation because its effects on hemodynamics are minimal. Etomidate inhibits adrenal mitochondrial hydroxylase activity and decreases steroidogenesis. Data suggest adrenal inhibition occurs even after one dose.[4] Because other agents can induce general anesthesia without producing adrenal insufficiency, etomidate should not be a first-line agent.

Ketamine, with its sympathomimetic properties and good analgesic effect, is sometimes used in the septic patient. Other positive properties of ketamine include stimulation of ventilation and bronchodilation. Salivary production increases with ketamine. If fiber-optic intubation is attempted, this increase in saliva may interfere with the laryngoscopic view of a difficult airway. In a stressed patient, ketamine's negative inotropic effects are unmasked as the patient's circulating catecholamines are depleted.[5] Ketamine induction is also associated with increased intracranial pressure, a consideration in patients with baseline elevated intracranial pressure. This may be mitigated by hyperventilation or by coadministering a benzodiazepine or propofol.

The systemic vasodilation and negative inotropy of induction agents, such as propofol[6,7] or thiopental, can be mitigated by pretreatment with an alpha-1 agonist or a beta agonist. Although cardiac output may increase with sepsis, the circulation of the induction agent is less predictable because of slower peripheral blood circulation. This may prolong the time for the intubating dose to take effect. At the same time, patient sensitivity is enhanced. The risk of overdosage and hemodynamic compromise thus increase. Transit time to effect is shorter with central access for induction than with peripheral access; central catheters, when available, should be the preferred routes for intravenous induction.

In cases of ileus, gastroparesis, or bowel obstruction, a classic rapid sequence induction may be preferred. Rapid sequence induction, however, obligates the anesthesiologist to a single predetermined drug dose, which may have unanticipated consequences in an already hemodynamically challenged patient. Another induction option that preserves hemodynamics and ventilation is the application of concentrated lidocaine to the airway. This option may be sufficient for septic patients, especially those with encephalopathy, as they may be amnestic and unaware even when little or no intravenous medication is given.

MONITORING THE SEPTIC PATIENT

Although not a single monitor has been proven to decrease patient mortality, the septic patient often leaves the operating room with more lines than limbs. The wide shifts in fluid volume and acute alterations in blood pressure in a septic patient frequently require invasive monitoring for quick diagnosis of hemodynamic changes.

Septic patients with ventilation/perfusion (V/Q) mismatch may need titrated ventilator support. Blood gases can be monitored after placement of arterial lines. Acid/base status, serum glucose, and electrolyte levels should be measured. When large quantities of fluids have been administered, blood pressure, hemoglobin, and changes in hematocrit in response to blood loss and blood transfusion also must be monitored. Rapid feedback of blood pressure changes can be essential to the titration of therapies in an unstable patient.

A single measurement of CVP, which is particularly poor in sepsis, is not a good indicator of volume status. With hypotension, a low CVP can be attributed to decreased intravascular volume, but a high CVP is not always the result of excess filling.[8] Other markers of volume status are blood pressure, response to fluid challenge, and systolic pressure variation (SPV). SPV on an arterial line tracing may suggest hypotension that is volume responsive. Thus, SPV greater than 10 mm Hg suggests adding fluids will increase blood pressure.[9] Decreased ventricular compliance, increased intrathoracic pressures from mechanical ventilation, and pulmonary hypertension may cause false CVP elevation.[8] Intravenous fluid administered through the central line can also alter CVP measurements. Recognizing the trend of CVP measurements and empirically administering fluids to see if increased preload helps blood pressure and hemodynamics can be beneficial.

Placing a pulmonary artery catheter (PAC) may be useful for a patient with uncertain cardiovascular status. A PAC is placed to measure continuous cardiac output and pulmonary artery pressure. By design, the PAC provides more useful data on the right ventricle than on the left. Mixed venous oxygen can be measured to determine oxygen delivery and consumption. In patients with severe pulmonary edema, it is the PAC which can help distinguish cardiogenic from noncardiogenic causes. The PAC may prompt a quick response by the physician to hemodynamic changes and to the effects of therapeutic intervention whether with volume expansion, diuresis, or titration of vasoactive drugs.[10] Specific risks associated with placement of a PAC include pulmonary artery rupture, ventricular arrhythmias, and even complete heart block if the patient has preexisting right bundle branch block. Patients with electrolyte disturbances, acidosis, and myocardial infarction are at risk for abnormal cardiac rhythms from the PAC, yet this is the population in which the catheter would more likely be placed.[11]

After the risks and benefits are weighed, the PAC should be considered in the patient who is unresponsive to standard therapy. Prognosis was improved in a subset of patients with circulatory shock when hemodynamic data prompted therapeutic changes.[10] Familiarity with the PAC likely improves its efficacy.[12]

NEUROMUSCULAR BLOCKADE AND SEPSIS

Sepsis alters the response to neuromuscular blockade. Nevertheless, these drugs can be an important part of the therapy for a septic patient. Aside from optimizing intubating conditions, they facilitate mechanical ventilation by keeping the patient's breathing synchronous with the ventilator, which increases lung compliance and decreases lung collapse. Neuromuscular blockade also minimizes excess oxygen consumption by reducing patient movement, especially respiratory movement.

Although very useful for rapid intubation, administration of succinylcholine can produce a massive hyperkalemic response,[13] which leads to wide complex bradycardia, ventricular arrhythmias, and ultimately cardiac arrest.[14] This risk is substantially higher 48 to 72 hours after onset of trauma, burns, and critical illness. Hyperkalemia has followed succinylcholine administration in patients with profound hemorrhage, metabolic acidosis, severe intra-abdominal infections,[14,15] and myopathy caused by steroids or immobilization.[16] For cardiac arrhythmias or arrest, cardiopulmonary resuscitation should be initiated and intravenous medications (calcium, bicarbonate, insulin, glucose, catecholamines) administered to acutely decrease serum potassium until the hyperkalemic episode resolves (10–20 minutes) and the patient is no longer resistant to defibrillation.[15]

Patients who are hypermetabolic have enhanced elimination kinetics that cause resistance to non-depolarizing muscle blockers (NDMB).[16] Increased alpha-1 acid glycoprotein binds NDMB and reduces free plasma concentrations of these relaxants, requiring increased induction doses. Termination of a single dose of NDMB is by redistribution from the neuromuscular junction.

Muscle relaxants have primarily hepatic metabolism and renal excretion. In sepsis, there is multi–organ system failure. With repeat injections of muscle relaxant, active metabolites (from rocuronium, pancuronium, and vecuronium) may accumulate, causing prolonged paralysis. Initial dosing may be increased in sepsis because of increased volume of distribution, even in the presence of kidney and liver dysfunction, but recovery from the paralytic may be prolonged or there may be a decreased need for redosing. Frequent monitoring of the train-of-four will help guide redosing of muscle relaxants.

LUNG INJURY

The septic patient often has a hospital course complicated by shock, lung injury, increased total body oxygen consumption, and prolonged dependence on a ventilator. Consequences of controlled ventilation, pain, and septic lung injury are increased V/Q mismatch, lung collapse, shunt, and dead space. The lung injury pattern can be heterogenous and lead to difficulty with mechanical ventilation. Larger tidal volumes will decrease lung collapse, but cause excess aerated lung distension. This contributes to worsening lung injury and the release of systemic inflammatory mediators. The degree of lung injury is frequently estimated by the amount of inspired oxygen support required to maintain adequate oxygen saturation. Acute lung injury is defined as the ratio of arterial oxygen concentration to fractional inspired oxygen (Pao_2/Fio_2) less than 300; in the acute respiratory distress syndrome the ratio is less than 200. In both conditions, there is four-quadrant airspace opacity, evidence of a low or normal left atrial pressure, and an inciting event.

When a patient is breathing spontaneously, intermittent deep breaths reinflate the lungs.[17] On mechanical ventilation, the shunt from lung collapse may be reversed by intermittent hyperinflation, such as achieved by maintaining a pressure of 30 cm H_2O for 30 seconds to reinflate atelectatic alveoli and improve V/Q matching. Some form of hyperinflation is often effective in the operating room to recruit alveoli and improve V/Q matching in a hypoxemic patient who does not respond to other ventilation methods. However, hyperinflation may cause barotrauma, and can decrease preload, resulting in profound hypotension.

Ventilation strategies to protect the lungs include the use of low tidal volumes (6 mL per ideal body weight in kilograms, plateau pressure $\leq$30 cm H_2O), permissive hypercapnia, and, more controversially, high positive end-expiratory pressure. With permissive hypercapnia and low tidal volumes, mortality and the number of ventilator-dependent days were decreased for patients with acute lung injury or respiratory distress syndrome.[18] Respiratory acidosis from ventilation at low tidal volumes can be compensated for by increasing the respiratory rate. Fio_2 is then titrated to adequate Pao_2 levels. Minimizing Fio_2 may help avoid oxygen toxicity, which could further worsen lung injury.

The reduced lung compliance associated with acute respiratory distress syndrome may dictate the use of an ICU ventilator in the operating room to manage lung injury in critical illness.[19] Older operating room ventilators are unable to maintain inspiratory flows at high pressures. At higher inspiratory flows and respiratory rates, ICU ventilators maintain minute ventilation, a difference that may be critical for the care of a patient with severely decreased lung compliance and impaired V/Q matching.

HEPATIC FAILURE

Patients with preoperative hepatic failure are at a substantially increased risk of perioperative mortality. In sepsis, changes in hepatic function are common. Although ischemia is a frequent cause of liver failure in the septic patient, especially when prolonged periods of hypotension require vasoactive support, hepatic function changes even in the absence of ischemia. Proteolysis, glycogenolysis, and gluconeogenesis are increased as part of a syndrome of muscle wasting, partial insulin resistance, and hyperglycemia. Bilirubin excretion is frequently altered; many patients manifest an elevated bilirubin, and the significance of this is unknown. Albumin levels decline while acute-phase proteins increase, leading to decreased plasma colloidal pressure, anasarca, and altered drug distribution. As always, the anesthesiologist should emphasize organ perfusion and prevention of aspiration, while also maintaining awareness of the potential for elevation of intracranial pressure, excess bleeding, and hypoglycemia.

Patients with preexisting hepatic pathology are at greater risk for fulminant hepatic failure than are other septic patients. When hepatic failure occurs, the first signs are metabolic and coagulation derangements. Both can be severe. Altered ammonia metabolism[20] can elevate intracranial pressure, causing ischemia and brain herniation. Hyponatremia and hyperglycemia can exacerbate intracranial hypertension.[21]

Treatment is targeted to reduce ammonia levels with lactulose and to decrease intracranial pressure with hyperventilation, mannitol, or propofol. Lactulose therapy can cause intravascular volume depletion and distend the abdomen, placing the patient at high risk for aspiration. Hypoglycemia, from reduced insulin metabolism and impaired gluconeogenesis, can also be life threatening. Hepatic encephalopathy can mask the clinical signs of hypoglycemia, so sugar levels should be checked frequently.

In the setting of hepatic dysfunction, larger initial doses of anesthetic may be needed; however, impaired metabolism will likely decrease the amount and need for frequent redosing. Short-acting opiates, such as fentanyl, can be titrated to produce analgesia. Morphine and meperidine are less suitable for septic patients because their metabolites have prolonged effects.

Coagulopathy is common with severe liver disease.[21,22] Hemostatic abnormalities can be attributed to platelet dysfunction and thrombocytopenia, decreased production of clotting factors, low fibrinogen levels, and low levels of vitamin K from malnutrition. Anemia is also common from gastrointestinal tract ulceration or bleeding varices. Laboratory values may show an elevated prothrombin time and international normalized ratio. Administration of vitamin K, an H_2 blocker, and possible replacement of clotting factors may be needed before an invasive procedure.

Patients with liver failure have poor splanchnic vasoregulation. Normally, the portal venous system acts as a variable-sized reservoir of blood volume to compensate for intravascular volume loss. With liver failure, especially when complicated by portal hypertension, this reserve is lost and the body may show less tolerance to hypovolemia.

RENAL FAILURE

Renal failure may result from sepsis as a consequence of decreased cardiac output, renal vasoconstriction, and renal tubule cellular dysfunction. Ideally, acute kidney injury is prevented by maintaining stable hemodynamics and avoiding known nephrotoxins, such as nonsteroidal anti-inflammatory drugs and aminoglycosides. Renal failure is prognostically very significant. If kidney injury in critically ill patients is severe enough to require dialysis, mortality rates can increase to more than 50%.[23]

Many therapies have been tested to prevent renal failure. Results have been limited. The effectiveness of diuretics,[24,25] sodium bicarbonate,[26] N-acetylcysteine,[27] dopamine,[28] or fenoldopam[29] to limit renal failure is inconclusive. Oliguria in the operating room is not abnormal, even in healthy subjects, and does not necessarily imply renal hypoperfusion.[30] Moreover, urine output is a poor marker of renal health, and measures to increase it may cause harm without benefit. Thus, the administration of diuretics to generate urine production does not improve renal function and may be detrimental.

The presence of renal dysfunction may inform extubation decisions. Because the kidney clears naturally occurring acids, metabolic acidosis is common. With metabolic acidosis, patients will hyperventilate to maintain a normal serum pH. Critical illness and surgery can make breathing and maintaining increased minute ventilation difficult. This may result in hypoventilation, worsening acidosis, obtundation, and cardiovascular compromise. In the face of uncertainty, leaving the acidemic patient with renal failure intubated after surgery may be safer.

Should surgery be delayed for dialysis in a patient with renal failure? Ideally, electrolytes, especially potassium, should be in a normal range before surgery. In the emergent situation, an arterial blood gas and potassium level should be obtained before surgery. In the setting of emergent surgery, electrolytes can be replenished in the operating room. If feasible, dialysis may also be instituted during surgery. Even when the patient is anuric, volume replacement should be considered to account for blood loss, third spacing, and the effects of vasodilatation. Of all possible therapies, maintaining hemodynamics and perfusion to the kidneys preserves renal function.[31]

BLOOD TRANSFUSION

Anemia is common in sepsis. It results from blood loss, nutritional deficiencies, insufficient erythropoietin production, frequent blood draws, and poor iron use.[32,33] In the perioperative setting, it is not always clear when and for what purpose to transfuse. Transfusion of packed red blood cells to obtain hemoglobin levels that match levels in healthy controls is not indicated in the septic patient. Blood products carry both infectious[34] and noninfectious risks,[35] including transfusion errors, anaphylaxis, transfusion-related acute lung injury, immunomodulation,[32] fever, nosocomial infection,[36] and coagulopathy ranging from hemolysis to disseminated intravascular coagulation.

Although blood products can be used as blood volume expanders, their use should also ideally target coagulation factor repletion or increased oxygen-carrying capacity. The benefit of giving blood to increase oxygen-carrying capacity is reduced by the effects of storage on packed red blood cells. Red cells stored for more than 15 days are not as efficient at releasing oxygen to tissues because of depletion of 2,3-diphosphoglycerate and decreased deformability, which causes microvascular sludging and ischemia.[32] The increase in oxygen uptake after administration of stored packed red blood cells is negligible, except in severe cases of anemia.

One way to minimize the negative effects associated with blood transfusion is to adopt a restrictive transfusion strategy and to give less blood. When transfusion was restricted to patients with hemoglobin levels below 7.0 g/dL, organ dysfunction, mortality, and ICU length of stay were comparable to those for patients whose hemoglobin levels were maintained above 10.0 g/dL.[37] Exceptions were patients with cardiovascular disease. The number of packed red blood cell units transfused independently predicts a worse clinical outcome.[38] A high study-exclusion rate and a low incidence of cardiovascular comorbidities limit the applicability of these findings. Leukocyte-depleted packed red blood cells, however, did reduce postoperative mortality when given to a subset of cardiac surgery patients.[39] Modern red cell units are frequently leukoreduced. The use of such units and the selective use of fresher red cell products might favor higher transfusion thresholds.

COLLOID VERSUS CRYSTALLOID

Septic patients frequently require large intravenous fluid resuscitations. Which fluid to use is a subject of debate. In healthy, unstressed patients, colloid normally increases intravascular oncotic pressure and pulls fluid from the interstitial space, thereby increasing intravascular volume. In the septic patient, colloid behaves differently because of greater capillary permeability that lets the colloid leak out. It may not be as effective.

In a large, randomized, controlled trial evaluating crystalloid and colloid in septic patients, no change was seen in 28-day mortality, requirements for mechanical ventilation, renal replacement therapy, or time in the ICU.[40] Outcomes of resuscitation were similar with colloid and crystalloid irrespective of baseline serum albumin levels.[41] Although colloid may help restore volume, using albumin does not reduce the risk of dying, and is more expensive than crystalloid.[42] Hydroxyethyl starches are a less-expensive colloid plasma substitute, but can cause coagulopathy, renal damage, and analyphalactoid reactions.[43]

Much ambiguity in the crystalloid and colloid literature may relate to the more important issue of the timing and intensity of resuscitation. The volume and time in which the fluid is given might be more important than the type of volume administered. Many other variables, such as vasoactive support, concomitant administration of blood products, and concentration of albumin (4%, 5%, or 25%) may also influence outcomes.

If a particular benefit to colloid resuscitation exists, it might be when hypotension must be reversed rapidly since a smaller volume of colloid than crystalloid is needed to achieve a similar effect. A small bolus challenge of colloid can help diagnose hypotension that is volume responsive. Other indications when colloid may be warranted include hypotension in a patient who is undergoing hemodialysis and for whom short-term volume shifts might be beneficial to facilitate fluid removal for intravascular volume expansion after large-volume paracentesis.[44] Colloid may also be warranted during the resolving phase of the acute respiratory distress syndrome.[45]

SODIUM BICARBONATE IN TREATING ACIDOSIS

Patients with sepsis are frequently acidemic. Carbon dioxide from a hypermetabolic catabolic state, lactate generation, and electrolyte abnormalities contribute to acidemia. It is the source of the acidemia, more than the pH, that is ominous. If electrolyte abnormalities are caused by renal tubular acidosis or diarrhea, then correction of the electrolyte imbalance with exogenous sodium bicarbonate may be effective. If lactic acidosis is caused by septic shock, however, the pH-altering effects of sodium bicarbonate last a short time, and the underlying source of acidosis remains.[46]

Because defibrillation may be more effective if the patient is not severely acidemic, administration of sodium bicarbonate in code situations may bring about the patient's responsiveness. Acidemia has negative inotropic effects.[47] It decreases beta cardiac receptors, response to catecholamines, and contractile function. It may, however, be protective by keeping the oxygen dissociation curve shifted to the right, helping hemoglobin more readily release oxygen to tissues. Although sodium bicarbonate often temporarily reverses the hemodynamic instability in acidosis, it may actually worsen the clinical picture by decreasing intracellular pH.

Bicarbonate is metabolized to water and carbon dioxide. Without a ventilation strategy to remove it, this excess carbon dioxide can worsen acidemia. Hypocalcemia, associated with bicarbonate infusion,[46,47] may worsen hemodynamics, and the alkalosis-associated left shift of the hemoglobin dissociation curve may worsen lactic acidosis because hemoglobin holds oxygen with greater affinity. Effective treatment of lactic acidosis depends on correcting its underlying cause.

GLYCEMIC CONTROL

Glucose variation is attributable to many factors: the patient's nutritional state, liver function, endogenous insulin supply, the stress response, and illness severity. Glucose levels fluctuate in critical illness and with circadian rhythms.[48] Anesthetized patients are less likely to show signs or symptoms of glucose level extremes. Their glucose levels should therefore be monitored frequently. Because glucometers vary in reliability, arterial glucose measurements give more accurate serum glucose values to guide therapy.

Of the many studies of glycemic control, two sentinel papers with conflicting outcomes have driven controversy. In 2001, Van den Berghe and colleagues[49] randomly assigned patients in a mostly cardiothoracic ICU to intensive insulin therapy versus less strict control, demonstrating a reduction in mortality, organ dysfunction, and ICU length of stay with tight glucose regulation from 80 to 110 mg/dL. In contrast, the NICE-SUGAR (Normoglycemia in Intensive Care Evaluation—Survival Using Glucose Algorithm Regulation) study in 2009 demonstrated no benefit with intensive insulin therapy and actually found increased mortality in the intensive insulin therapy group.[50] There were many differences in these two studies which make it difficult to conclude the optimal glycemic therapy for septic ICU patients.

However, some other findings have shown some consistency. For example, a single episode of hypoglycemia with glucose less than 40 mg/dL has been correlated with increased mortality[51]; this prompted the early termination of two large trials.[52,53] Insulin dose[54] and blood glucose variability have also been found to be independent correlates for increased mortality.[55,56]

The perfect blood sugar level for a septic patient remains unknown. Intensive insulin therapy to maintain glucose levels from 80 to 110 mg/dL can result in hypoglycemic episodes. Glucose levels greater than 180 mg/dL have the adverse effects of osmotic diuresis and protein glycosylation. Therefore, the ideal glucose level may be somewhere between these points. Also, since insulin dose has been correlated with increased mortality, it may be better to minimize parenteral glucose in total parenteral nutrition and dextrose-containing infusions while administering insulin as a way to decrease exogenous insulin requirements.

ADRENAL INSUFFICIENCY IN SEPTIC SHOCK

In a hemodynamically unstable patient, hypotension may be caused by adrenal insufficiency. If a patient's use of steroids has been greater than 5 mg/d for more than 3 weeks in the past year,[57] steroid replacement may be needed. Exogenous administration of steroids is associated with protein catabolism, insulin resistance,[58] immunosuppression, and leukocytosis that may delay the diagnosis of an infection. Adrenal insufficiency may be diagnosed by symptoms or by laboratory values. Hypotension that is refractory to resuscitation may indicate adrenal insufficiency. For a positive diagnosis of adrenal insufficiency in the septic patient, suggested diagnostic thresholds include a baseline cortisol that is less than 15 μg/dL or a change of 9 μg/dL from baseline in response to adrenocorticotrophic hormone stimulation.[59] The reliability of these values for diagnosing adrenal insufficiency has been questioned.

The effect of steroid replacement on mortality, time to reversal of shock,[60–62] and dosing varies. The hemodynamic effects of intravenous steroids may take 2 to 6 hours to become evident, so alternative strategies may be necessary to resolve acute hemodynamic instability in the operating room. However, in the absence of laboratory values, replacement of steroids should be considered in patients with hypotension unresponsive to vasoactive agents and volume.

SUMMARY

Surgery in the septic patient is a rescue attempt. For the septic patient taken to surgery, death is a possible reality, not a rare chance. The decision to bring a septic patient to the operating room can be difficult. It requires the conviction that the planned intervention will correct an otherwise unacceptable trajectory. ICU care can help guide operating room decisions. The anesthesiologist must be vigilant in responding to rapidly changing physiology, the interplay between failing organ systems, and the dynamic balance between the beneficial and detrimental implications of every intervention. Although guided by critical care principles, anesthesiologists must give acute short-term goals priority over the long-term outcomes frequently used to justify therapies in the medical literature. Surviving the surgery is the important first priority of care.

REFERENCES

1. Marik PE, Varon J. The hemodynamic derangements in sepsis: implications for treatment strategies. Chest 1998;114:854–60.
2. Rivers E, Nguyen B, Havstad S, et al. Early goal-directed therapy in the treatment of severe sepsis and septic shock. N Engl J Med 2001;345:1368–77.
3. Roberts JA, Lipman J. Pharmacokinetic issues for antibiotics in the critically ill patient. Crit Care Med 2009;37:840–51.
4. Hildreth AN, Mejia VA, Maxwell RA, et al. Adrenal suppression following a single dose of etomidate for rapid sequence induction: a prospective randomized study. J Trauma 2008;65:573–9.
5. Sinner B, Graf BM. Ketamine. Handb Exp Pharmacol 2008;182:313–33.
6. Vasile B, Rasulo F, Candiani A, et al. The pathophysiology of propofol infusion syndrome: a simple name for a complex syndrome. Intensive Care Med 2003;29:1417–25.
7. Fudickar A, Bein B. Propofol infusion syndrome: update of clinical manifestation and pathophysiology. Minerva Anestesiol 2009;75:339–44.
8. Magder S, Bafaqeeh F. The clinical role of central venous pressure measurements. J Intensive Care Med 2007;22:44–51.
9. Barbeito A, Mark JB. Arterial and central venous pressure monitoring. Anesthesiol Clin 2006;24:717–35.
10. Mimoz O, Rauss A, Rekik N, et al. Pulmonary artery catheterization in critically ill patients: a prospective analysis of outcome changes associated with catheter-prompted changes in therapy. Crit Care Med 1994;22:573–9.
11. Matthay MA, Chatterjee K. Bedside catheterization of the pulmonary artery: risks compared with benefits. Ann Intern Med 1988;109:826–34.
12. Iberti TJ, Fischer EP, Leibowitz AB, et al. A multicenter study of physicians' knowledge of the pulmonary artery catheter. Pulmonary artery catheter study group. JAMA 1990;264:2928–32.
13. Markewitz BA, Elstad MR. Succinylcholine-induced hyperkalemia following prolonged pharmacologic neuromuscular blockade. Chest 1997;111:248–51.
14. Matthews JM. Succinylcholine-induced hyperkalemia and rhabdomyolysis in a patient with necrotizing pancreatitis. Anesth Analg 2000;91:1552–4.
15. Kohlschutter B, Baur H, Roth F. Suxamethonium-induced hyperkalaemia in patients with severe intra-abdominal infections. Br J Anaesth 1976;48:557–62.
16. Jeevendra Martyn JA, Fukushima Y, Chon JY, et al. Muscle relaxants in burns, trauma, and critical illness. Int Anesthesiol Clin 2006;44(2):123–43.
17. Bendixen HH, Hedley-Whyte J, Laver MB. Impaired oxygenation in surgical patients during general anesthesia with controlled ventilation. N Engl J Med 1963;269:991–6.
18. The Acute Respiratory Distress Syndrome Network. Ventilation with lower tidal volumes as compared with traditional tidal volumes for acute lung injury and the acute respiratory distress syndrome. N Engl J Med 2000;342:1301–8.
19. Tung A, Drum ML, Morgan S. Effect of inspiratory time on tidal volume delivery in anesthesia and intensive care unit ventilators operating in pressure control mode. Clin Anesth 2005;17:8–15.
20. Clay AS, Hainline BE. Hyperammonemia in the ICU. Chest 2007;132:1368–78.
21. Stravitz RT, Kramer AH, Davern T, et al. Intensive care of patients with acute liver failure: recommendations of the U.S. Acute Liver Failure Study Group. Crit Care Med 2007;35:2498–508.

22. Stravitz RT. Critical management decisions in patients with acute liver failure. Chest 2008;134:1092–102.
23. Cho KC, Himmelfarb J, Paganini E, et al. Survival by dialysis modality in critically ill patients with acute kidney injury. J Am Soc Nephrol 2006;17:3132–8.
24. Sampath S, Moran JL, Graham PL. The efficacy of loop diuretics in acute renal failure: assessment using Bayesian evidence synthesis techniques. Crit Care Med 2007;35:2516–24.
25. Karajala V, Mansour W, Kellum JA. Diuretics in acute kidney injury. Minerva Anestesiol 2009;75:251–7.
26. Weisberg LS. Sodium bicarbonate for renal protection after heart surgery: Let's wait and see. Crit Care Med 2009;37:333–4.
27. Naughton F, Wijeysundera D, Karkouti K, et al. N-acetylcysteine to reduce renal failure after cardiac surgery: a systematic review and meta-analysis. Can J Anaesth 2008;55:827–35.
28. Ichai C, Soubielle J, Carles M, et al. Comparison of the renal effects of low to high doses of dopamine and dobutamine in critically ill patients: a single-blind randomized study. Crit Care Med 2008;28:921–8.
29. Landoni G, Biondi-Zoccai GG, Tumlin JA, et al. Beneficial impact of fenoldopam in critically ill patients with or at risk for acute renal failure: a meta-analysis of randomized clinical trials. Am J Kidney Dis 2007;49:56–68.
30. Alpert RA, Roizen MF, Hamilton WK, et al. Intraoperative urinary output does not predict postoperative renal function in patients undergoing abdominal aortic revascularization. Surgery 1984;95:707–11.
31. Brienza N, Giglio MT, Marucci M, et al. Does perioperative hemodynamic optimization protect renal function in surgical patients? A meta-analytic study. Crit Care Med 2009;37:2079–90.
32. Raghavan M, Marik PE. Anemia, allogenic blood transfusion, and immunomodulation in the critically ill. Chest 2005;127:295–307.
33. Vincent JL, Baron JF, Reinhart K, et al. Anemia and blood transfusion in critically ill patients. JAMA 2002;288:1499–507.
34. Wagner SJ. Transfusion-transmitted bacterial infections: risks, sources and interventions. Vox Sang 2004;86:157–63.
35. Hendrickson JE, Hillyer CD. Noninfectious serious hazards of transfusion. Anesth Analg 2009;108:759–69.
36. Taylor RW, Manganaro L, O'Brien J, et al. Impact of allogenic packed red blood cell transfusion on nosocomial infection rates in the critically ill patient. Crit Care Med 2002;30:2249–54.
37. Hebert PC, Well G, Blajchman MA, et al. A mulitcenter, randomized, controlled clinical trial of transfusion requirements in critical care. N Engl J Med 1999;340: 409–18.
38. Corwin HL, Gettinger A, Pearl RG, et al. The CRIT study: anemia and blood transfusion in the critically ill—current clinical practice in the United States. Crit Care Med 2004;32:39–52.
39. van de Watering LMG, Hermans J, Houbiers JGA, et al. Beneficial effects of leukocyte depletion of transfused blood on postoperative complications in patients undergoing cardiac surgery; a randomized clinical trial. Circulation 1998;97:562–8.
40. Finfer S, Bellomo R, Boyce N, et al. A comparison of albumin and saline for fluid resuscitation in the intensive care unit. N Engl J Med 2004;350: 2247–56.

41. Finfer S, Bellomo R, McEvoy S, et al. Effect of baseline serum albumin concentration on outcome of resuscitation with albumin or saline in patients in intensive care units: analysis of data from the saline versus albumin fluid evaluation (SAFE) study. BMJ 2006;333:1044.

42. Alderson P, Bunn F, Lefebvre C, et al. Human albumin solution for resuscitation and volume expansion in critically ill patients. Cochrane Database Syst Rev 2004;(4):CD001208.

43. Sakr Y, Payden D, Reinhart K, et al. Effects of hydroxyethyl starch administration on renal function in critically ill patients. Br J Anaesth 2007;98:216–24.

44. Fan E, Stewart TE. Albumin in critical care: SAFE, but worth its salt? Crit Care 2004;8:297–9.

45. Rivers EP. Fluid-management strategies in acute lung injury—liberal, conservative, or both? N Engl J Med 2006;354:2598–600.

46. Boyd JH, Walley KR. Is there a role for sodium bicarbonate in treating lactic acidosis from shock? Curr Opin Crit Care 2008;14:379–83.

47. Forsythe SM, Schmidt GA. Sodium bicarbonate for the treatment of lactic acidosis. Chest 2000;117:260–7.

48. Egi M, Bellomo R, Stachowski E, et al. Circadian rhythm of blood glucose values in critically ill patients. Crit Care Med 2007;35:416–21.

49. van den Berghe G, Wouters P, Weekers F, et al. Intensive insulin therapy in critically ill patients. N Engl J Med 2001;345:1359–67.

50. The NICE-SUGAR Study Investigators. Intensive versus conventional glucose control in critically ill patients. N Engl J Med 2009;360:1283–97.

51. Krinsley JS, Grover A. Severe hypoglycemia in critically ill patients: risk factors and outcomes. Crit Care Med 2007;35:2262–7.

52. Brunkhorst FM, Engel C, Bloos F, et al. Intensive insulin therapy and pentastarch resuscitation in severe sepsis. N Engl J Med 2008;358:125–39.

53. Preiser JC, Devos P, Ruiz-Santana S, et al. A prospective randomized multicentre controlled trial on tight glucose control by intensive insulin therapy in adult intensive care units: the Glucontrol Study. Intensive Care Med 2009;35:1738–48.

54. Finney SJ, Zekveld C, Elia A, et al. Glucose control and mortality in critically ill patients. JAMA 2003;290:2041–7.

55. Ali NA, O'Brien JM Jr, Dungan K, et al. Glucose variability and mortality in patients with sepsis. Crit Care Med 2008;36:2316–21.

56. Egi M, Bellomo R, Stachowski E, et al. Variability of blood glucose concentration and short-term mortality in critically ill patients. Anesthesiology 2006;105:244–52.

57. Salem M, Tainsh RE Jr, Bromberg J, et al. Perioperative glucocorticoid coverage. A reassessment 42 years after emergence of a problem. Ann Surg 1994;219: 416–25.

58. Bornstein SR. Predisposing factors for adrenal insufficiency. N Engl J Med 2009; 360:2328–39.

59. Lipiner-Friedman D, Srung CL, Laterre PF, et al. Adrenal function in sepsis: the retrospective Corticus Cohort Study. Crit Care Med 2007;35:1012–8.

60. Sprung CL, Annane D, Keh D, et al. Hydrocortisone therapy for patients with septic shock. N Engl J Med 2008;358:111–24.

61. Annane D, Bellissant E, Bollaert PE, et al. Corticosteroids for treating severe sepsis and septic shock. Cochrane Database Syst Rev 2004;(1):CD002243.

62. Annane D, Bellissant E, Bollaert PE, et al. Corticosteorids in the treatment of severe sepsis and septic shock in adults: a systematic review. JAMA 2009; 301:2361–75.

Anesthesia for Patients Requiring Advanced Ventilatory Support

James M. Blum, MD*, Ross Blank, MD, Lauryn R. Rochlen, MD

KEYWORDS

- ARDS • Respiratory failure • Ventilation
- Anesthesia • ECMO • HFOV

The critically ill patient who requires anesthesia is frequently a concern for the anesthesiologist. In addition to having potential hemodynamic lability and coagulopathy, the critically ill patient frequently experiences profound respiratory failure. The approach to the patient requiring advanced ventilatory support requires an understanding of respiratory failure, the pathophysiology causing respiratory failure and hypoxia, the physiology of mechanical ventilation and the advanced modes of ventilation available in the intensive care unit (ICU). Many of the modes available on ICU ventilators are not available or applicable to the operating room (OR), but being able to replicate them using similar settings is key to preserving acceptable oxygenation and avoiding ventilator-induced lung injury (VILI). This article discusses the basic definitions of hypoxia and common pathologic states, reviews the physiology of mechanical ventilation and advanced forms of ventilation available in the ICU, and concludes with recommendations for the management of patients with severe respiratory failure when they are taken to the OR.

DEFINITIONS AND PATHOLOGY

Respiratory failure has a multitude of causes and generally results in a combination of poor oxygenation and ventilation; however, oxygenation is the primary concern as hypercarbia is rarely life threatening and typically manageable. The definition of hypoxia is defined as an inadequate supply of oxygen. The quantification of hypoxia is more challenging. A widely accepted, yet controversial, method of quantifying hypoxemia is the A-a gradient, which is calculated by subtracting the amount of oxygen

Division of Critical Care Medicine, Department of Anesthesiology, University of Michigan Medical Center, University of Michigan Medical School, 1500 East Medical Center Drive, Ann Arbor, MI 48109, USA
* Corresponding author.
E-mail address: jmblum@umich.edu

Anesthesiology Clin 28 (2010) 25–38
doi:10.1016/j.anclin.2010.01.009
1932-2275/10/$ – see front matter © 2010 Elsevier Inc. All rights reserved.

dissolved in blood (Pa_{O_2}) from alveolar oxygen tension (PA_{O_2}).[1] The A-a gradient involves substantial arithmetic because calculating the PA_{O_2} requires the alveolar gas equation:

$$PA_{O_2} = (760 - 47) \times F_{IO_2} - Pa_{CO_2}/0.8$$

Hence, the Pa_{O_2}/F_{IO_2} (P/F ratio) has become a common method of describing hypoxia, and is used as a primary criterion in the definition of certain types of lung pathology.[2] A common concern of the A-a gradient and P/F ratio is the lack of incorporation of other parameters that affect oxygenation other than the F_{IO_2}. This has led to the development of the oxygenation index (OI):

$$OI = (F_{IO_2} \times mean\ airway\ pressure)/Pa_{O_2}$$

However, thus far, it has not been used as a primary measure in defining disease states.[3]

The pathology causing hypoxia is important as there are ventilator strategies that have been shown to provide improvement in long-term survival in acute lung injury (ALI) and acute respiratory distress syndrome (ARDS). The definitions of these disorders are shown in **Box 1**. In these disorders, the ARDSnet ARMA trial showed that ventilation with 6 mL/kg predicted body weight (PBW) with ventilator plateau pressures <30 cm H_2O using a specifically prescribed positive end-expiratory pressure (PEEP) and F_{IO_2} reduced the likelihood of mortality.[4] These specific settings are available at http://www.ardsnet.org.

To date, there is a lack of large-scale, randomized trial data supporting survival benefits of other ventilation strategies in ALI/ARDS or other pathologies in the adult population. Despite this, it is commonly accepted that VILI affects long-term outcomes and occurs through a variety of methods including barotrauma (too much pressure applied to the lung), volutrauma (too much volume per breath), and atelectrauma (constant opening and closing of lung units).[5] This has promoted the use of open lung strategies (OLS) to prevent trauma to the lung while providing maximal oxygenation to the patient.[6] Many OLS are promoted, and many of these involve advanced ventilator modes. However, to understand these modes, one must comprehend the basic physiology of mechanical ventilation.

THE PHYSIOLOGY OF MECHANICAL VENTILATION
Mechanics

At its most basic level, mechanical ventilation is positive-pressure ventilation in which the ventilator creates positive pressure (relative to atmospheric pressure) at the airway opening. This results in the flow of gas from the airway opening to the lungs and an increase in the volume of the elastic respiratory system (lungs and chest wall). Positive-pressure ventilation is in contrast to spontaneous breathing during which the muscles of respiration create negative intrathoracic pressure. In mechanical and

Box 1
Definition of ARDS/ALI
Acute respiratory failure
Diffuse bilateral infiltrates on chest radiograph
Absence of left atrial hypertension
Hypoxemia (P/F ratio <200 for ARDS, P/F ratio <300 for ALI)

spontaneous ventilation, expiration is a passive process dependent on the elastic recoil of the respiratory system.

The interplay of pressure, flow, volume, and the mechanical properties of the respiratory system is summarized by the equation of motion:

$$\Delta Pressure = Flow \times Resistance + \Delta Volume/Compliance$$

In this equation, ΔPressure refers to the total pressure generated by the respiratory muscles and that applied to the airway opening. The equation shows that the total pressure can be divided into a component of airways resistance (Flow = ΔP/R by Ohm's Law) and an elastic component (Compliance = ΔV/ΔP = 1/Elastance). The relevant ΔV is the tidal volume (V_T).[7]

Monitoring patients during mechanical ventilation involves measuring pressure at the airway opening. There is no simple way to directly measure pressure in the alveoli or the likely more important transpulmonary pressure (defined as the difference in pressure from inside the alveolus to outside the alveolus; ie, in the pleural space).[8] This is shown in **Fig. 1**.

For patients who are deeply sedated and/or pharmacologically paralyzed, the contribution of the respiratory muscles is nil. In such cases, ΔP can be measured at the airway opening as peak inspiratory pressure (PIP) – end-expiratory pressure. When ventilator settings or expiratory mechanics lead to PEEP, ΔP becomes PIP – PEEP. Thus, rearranging the equation of motion gives

$$PIP = Flow \times R + V_T/C + PEEP$$

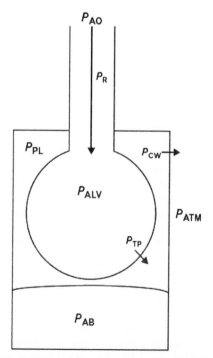

Fig. 1. Pressures in the respiratory system. (*From* Hess DR, Bigatello LM. The chest wall in acute lung injury/acute respiratory distress syndrome. Curr Opin Crit Care 2008;14:95; with permission.)

Thus, there are many possible causes for high PIPs during mechanical ventilation. Specifically, high inspiratory flow, high airways resistance, high tidal volume, low compliance, and high PEEP (either applied or intrinsic) can all contribute to high PIP.

In an effort to simplify the assessment of airway pressure, the equation of motion can be simplified by an end-inspiratory pause. During such a pause, the inspiratory and expiratory valves of the ventilator circuit close and gas flow ceases. The airway pressure drops to a plateau pressure less than PIP during this pause such that

$$\Delta Pressure = P_{PLAT} - PEEP = Flow \times R + V_T/C$$

$$P_{PLAT} - PEEP = V_T/C \text{ because Flow} = 0.$$

Determination of P_{PLAT} gives an approximation of alveolar pressure assuming that there is a static column of gas between the airway opening and the alveoli during the pause. It also allows for calculation of the compliance of the respiratory system. Accordingly, the difference between PIP and P_{PLAT} corresponds to the Flow $\times$ R term and allows for calculation of resistance for a given value of flow.

Management of Ventilation and Oxygenation

Management of ventilation and CO_2 clearance with mechanical ventilation is relatively straightforward. Minute ventilation is the product of tidal volume and respiratory rate and these 2 parameters can be directly controlled with older and newer operating room (OR) ventilators. Moreover, continuous monitoring of end-tidal CO_2 in the OR allows for real-time feedback on the adequacy of ventilation. Situations may arise during which CO_2 clearance is inadequate despite seemingly adequate minute ventilation. This situation may occur with increased CO_2 production (eg, sepsis, malignant hyperthermia) or increased dead space (eg, extensions of the breathing circuit distal to the Y-piece or abnormalities in the pulmonary circulation).

Traditional ventilator teaching stresses that F_{IO_2} and PEEP are the 2 primary variables that influence oxygenation. The former is intuitive and follows from the alveolar gas equation. The effect of PEEP is more complicated. The alveolar gas equation shows the factors that determine the partial pressure of oxygen in the alveolus but does not address how such oxygen enters the circulation. The latter process depends intimately on ventilation-perfusion (V/Q) matching. At one extreme, when V/Q = 0, blood flows from the right to the left side of the heart without encountering any ventilated alveoli. This situation, called shunt, always exists at a low level as a result of anatomic factors such as the bronchial and Thebesian circulations. Pathologic shunts include intracardiac right-to-left shunts, pulmonary arteriovenous malformations, and, most commonly, blood flow through poorly ventilated lung as seen in atelectasis, pneumonia, and pulmonary edema. At the other extreme, dead space, where V/Q approaches infinity, regions of the lungs are ventilated but not well perfused and minimal gas exchange can occur. In reality, the lungs constitute a heterogeneous collection of units with a spectrum of V/Q ratios that can be modified by mechanical ventilation.[7]

The intent of applied PEEP is to prevent cyclic atelectasis and maintain alveoli continuously above their respective closing pressures. When effective, this will reduce or eliminate regions of intrapulmonary shunt and improve V/Q matching and oxygenation. However, PEEP can paradoxically worsen oxygenation if regional over distention redistributes perfusion from high to low V/Q units. Also, the increase in pulmonary vascular resistance associated with high airway pressures may favor passage of blood through an intracardiac shunt and worsen oxygenation. Exactly how to apply PEEP and how much PEEP to apply remain controversial questions. Moreover, PEEP can have other adverse effects, namely an increase in intrathoracic pressure that limits venous return and barotrauma.[7]

A useful concept when considering the effects of PEEP and other ventilator settings on oxygenation is that of mean airway pressure (mPaw). The typical beneficial effect of PEEP on oxygenation may be attributed to an increase in mPaw that reduces intrapulmonary shunt. mPaw is simply the airway pressure averaged over the respiratory cycle. With conventional ventilator settings, PEEP largely determines mPaw because more time is spent in the expiratory than the inspiratory phase when the I/E ratio is ~1:2. Ventilator modes that maintain a high inspiratory pressure and lengthen the inspiratory time (and thus increase or invert the I/E ratio) result in a further elevation in mPaw. This is the basis of the further improvements in oxygenation that may be seen with advanced ventilatory modes. All the adverse effects noted for applied PEEP are also relevant to elevations in mPaw created by adjustments in ventilator settings.

In addition, adjustments that increase mPaw and thereby limit the expiratory time may increase the likelihood of intrinsic or auto-PEEP. Auto-PEEP refers to the persistence of expiratory flow (and therefore of an expiratory pressure > the applied PEEP) when the patient or ventilator initiates the next inspiration. Auto-PEEP is commonly seen in patients with obstructive lung disease who exhibit delayed expiration. Auto-PEEP can also be induced in patients with or without obstructive disease when they are subjected to rapid respiratory rates, high tidal volumes, and/or shortened expiratory times. For a patient on a mechanical ventilator, auto-PEEP is most easily detected by observation of the flow versus time waveform and evidence that expiratory flow does not return to zero before the subsequent inspiration. Auto-PEEP can be measured during an end-expiratory pause. During volume-control ventilation (VCV), auto-PEEP may be detected by a progressive increase in PIP caused by progressive hyperinflation. During pressure-controlled ventilation (PCV), there will be a progressive loss of tidal volume as the PIP is fixed. Auto-PEEP may also prevent ventilator triggering by not allowing patients to generate the negative pressure or inward flow necessary to open the inspiratory valve in modes that allow for spontaneous breaths. Most importantly, auto-PEEP can aggravate the deleterious hemodynamic and barotraumatic effects of applied PEEP and mPaw caused by further increase of intrathoracic pressures.[7]

ADVANCED MODES OF VENTILATION

When deciding which mode of ventilatory support to apply to a hypoxic patient, it is vital to keep in mind that responses are not always predictable and may be highly variable between patients. This is particularly true for the patient in respiratory failure with other comorbidities and concomitant organ dysfunction. It is important to monitor the patient's response to a particular ventilator setting by continued assessment of pulmonary compliance and serial arterial blood gases. Patients with respiratory failure who are difficult to ventilate and oxygenate on conventional VCV modes may benefit from PCV in which strict pressure limitation can be achieved. With close monitoring of VCV, similar results to PCV can be obtained; however, advanced ventilators with servo-controlled valves are able to provide additional control and volumes at lower pressures not obtainable with VCV.

PCV

Features specific to pressure-controlled modes contribute to improved gas exchange and patient-ventilator interaction.[9] The most basic settings of this mode include a respiratory rate, FIO_2, PEEP, drive pressure (ΔP), and I/E ratio. Inspiration can be pressure or time cycled. Tidal volumes are generated by the pressure difference achieved from beginning to end of inspiration and vary with the airway resistance and compliance. The inspiratory time is determined by the clinician and can be adjusted based on the patient's lung mechanics. A large portion of tidal volume is delivered early in the cycle resulting in higher average mPaw compared with VCV, although adjusting the flow rate and using additional ventilator settings may reduce this increase and result in lower pressures for equal tidal volumes.

PCV offers several advantages for the patient in severe respiratory failure. The concept of pressure-limited ventilation maintains PIP less than a specified value, decreasing the risk of macro- and microscopic barotraumas. The decelerating flow pattern of PCV produces a more uniform distribution of ventilation with the lung fields, which is beneficial in heterogeneous lungs. Another potential benefit of the decelerating flow pattern is that most of the tidal volume is delivered early on in inspiration. This provides higher mPaw over the course of the respiratory cycle. Higher mPaw results in improved oxygenation.[10,11]

PCV may be especially beneficial in patients with ALI and ARDS. The variable flow rates used in PCV improve patient work of breathing and limit high PIP. The increased mPaw leads to improves oxygenation, which is often difficult in these patients. Shorter expiration times may lead to increased auto-PEEP, which can also lead to improved oxygenation.

The disadvantages and limitations of using PCV also warrant discussion. Improvement in oxygenation from an increase in mPaw depends on the amount of lung tissue available for recruitment. In highly damaged and inflamed lung in which compliance is poor, it is difficult to achieve adequate ventilation while maintaining pressure limits. When lung damage is heterogeneous, normal lung regions may be overinflated and at risk for VILI. Maximum flow rates early during inspiration expose the distal airways to high shearing, also increasing the risk of VILI. As lung compliance improves, PCV provides a mechanism for the introduction of volutrauma if the ventilator settings are not changed.

Airway Pressure Release Ventilation and Biphasic Positive Airway Pressure

Quests to improve oxygenation, pulmonary mechanics and reduce VILI have led to the development of more advanced modes of ventilation that can commonly be seen in use in ICUs. Two such modes are airway pressure release ventilation (APRV) and biphasic positive airway pressure (BIPAP). Both modes are extensions of PCV that exhibit similar concepts and physiology as PCV. These modes are typically reserved for patients with difficult to manage ALI or ARDS, and their implementation is often limited by lack of clinician comfort and knowledge with managing the ventilator settings and potential patient-ventilator interactions and patient responses.

Barriers to using APRV or BIPAP may be related to confusion regarding the definitions and parameters of these 2 modes, which may differ between institutions due to branding by ventilator companies. A review of definitional criteria by Rose and Hawkins,[12] which examined 50 studies and 18 discussion articles investigating APRV and/or BIPAP, revealed discrepancies in the descriptions of APRV and BIPAP.

Such ambiguity makes the use and discussion of these modes difficult and often frustrating. They found that further confusion is caused by ventilator branding and reference terms for ventilator setup. This study found that APRV and BIPAP are described in the literature as the same mode, on a continuum, or as distinctively different modes. The major distinction between modes found in this review was the mean duration of expiration time, which was approximately 3 times longer in BIPAP compared with APRV (**Fig. 2**). Inspiratory pressure (P_{high}) and expiratory pressure (P_{low}) were reported as similar for either mode.

Original descriptions of these modes were published within 2 years of each other. APRV was first described in 1987 by Stock and Downs[13] from the United States

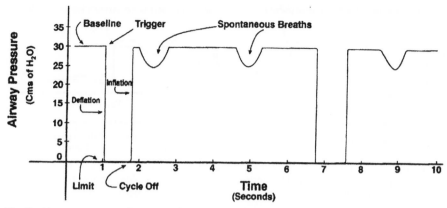

Fig. 2. Airway pressure release ventilation. (*From* Frawley PM, Habashi NM. Airway pressure release ventilation: theory and practice. AACN Clin Issues 2001;12(2):235; with permission.)

and was described as continuous positive airway pressure (CPAP) with an intermittent release phase. BIPAP was then described in 1989 by the European team of Baum and colleagues[14] as a mode that combined PCV with spontaneous ventilation.

APRV and BIPAP are both pressure-limited, time-cycled modes (**Figs. 3** and **4**).[15] The basic settings are similar to those of PCV; however, instead of the drive pressure being set, a high pressure P_{high} (ie, PIP) and a low pressure P_{low} (ie, PEEP) are set. Ventilation occurs by alternating between 2 pressure levels, P_{high} and P_{low}. A key difference between these modes and PCV is that these modes allow for spontaneous breathing independent of ventilator cycling using an active inspiratory valve. A spontaneous breath can be taken by the patient at any point in the respiratory cycle. If the patient is not breathing spontaneously, both modes are virtually identical to conventional PCV, perhaps with an extended I time. The degree of ventilatory support is determined by time spent at both pressure levels and the subsequent tidal volume achieved. As mentioned earlier, the primary distinction between modes is that there are no restrictions on the duration of time spent at P_{low}, or release pressure in APRV. Original descriptions of APRV used durations of P_{low} less than or equal to

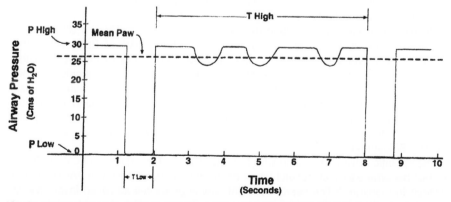

Fig. 3. Airway pressure release ventilation. (*From* Frawley PM, Habashi NM. Airway pressure release ventilation: theory and practice. AACN Clin Issues 2001;12(2):238; with permission.)

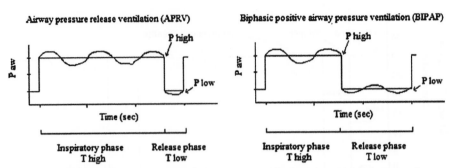

Fig. 4. APRV and BIPAP airway pressure tracings. (*From* Seymour CW, Frazer M, Reilly PM, et al. Airway pressure release and biphasic intermittent positive airway pressure ventilation: are they ready for prime time? J Trauma 2007;62(5):1300; with permission.)

1.5 seconds.[13] The time spent at P_{low} (T_{low}) is set for adequate carbon dioxide removal, and not so long as to lead to de-recruitment. P_{low} can be titrated exactly like PEEP to be maintained higher than the lower inflection point on the compliance curve, allowing for optimal lung mechanics.

One of the major advantages of APRV and BIPAP is improved distribution of gas to dependent regions of the lung as a result of the effects of spontaneous ventilation, leading to improved V/Q matching.[16] This is caused by movement of posterior sections of the diaphragm that occurs during spontaneous ventilation, but is absent during mechanical breaths. In addition, spontaneous ventilation reduces the amount of positive-pressure ventilation required during the respiratory cycle, which can result in improved hemodynamics by reducing the negative cardiovascular effects of positive pressure. There is also evidence supporting an increase in glomerular filtration rate and sodium excretion, as well as improved liver function as a result of spontaneous ventilation.[15] Patients with left ventricular dysfunction may not tolerate the increased preload and left ventricular afterload that accompanies spontaneous breaths. Although hemodynamic instability may be disadvantageous in certain patient populations, there are no absolute contraindications to using APRV or BIPAP.

Another proposed advantage is improved patient-ventilator interaction. Dyssynchrony may increase the work of breathing, leading to an increase in oxygen consumption and reductions in effective ventilatory support. Improved synchrony with the ventilator results in decreased need for sedation and neuromuscular blockade, another potential advantage.[15,17]

Despite the evidence supporting the beneficial effects of APRV and BIPAP, there are also questions that remain to be answered in future trials.[17] Suggestions that spontaneous breaths taken while at higher pressure levels may result in even higher inflation volumes and pressure, aggravating VILI need to be examined further. There are also some who question the need for less sedation and neuromuscular blockade as some data suggest patients with severe ARDS should not breath spontaneously. One major outstanding concern is how to standardize the application of APRV and BIPAP to assist clinicians in determining optimal settings and making adjustments.

The specific advantages seen with the application of inverse ratio PCV, APRV, or BIPAP become especially useful when caring for the patient with ALI/ARDS that is difficult to manage.[18] The nearly constant airway pressures achieved favor alveolar recruitment, which should improve oxygenation. Short expiratory times promote ventilation in healthier alveoli, again increasing oxygenation and V/Q matching. Some

arguments for spontaneous ventilation can also be extrapolated to this patient population. Lower requirements for sedation may be beneficial because of decreased
effects of sedating medications on other organ functions and less accumulation.
Minimal sedation will also allow acute complications, such as changes in mental
status, to be more easily recognized. The avoidance of neuromuscular blockade
reduces the likelihood of myopathy of critical illness. Despite these potential benefits,
there is no large-scale randomized data suggesting improved long-term outcomes
from the use of any of the ventilatory modes.

High-Frequency Oscillatory Ventilation

High-frequency oscillatory ventilation (HFOV) works by providing exceptionally
small tidal volumes at a high mPaw,[19] which is believed to be lung protective
as it avoids the atelectrauma from other higher volume forms of ventilation and
maintains open lung to help improve oxygenation. HFOV is similar to other forms
of jet ventilation, but in HFOV, there is an active expiratory component that
improves ventilation.[20]

HFOV devices operate with a continuous flow of fresh gas (bias flow) of 30 to 60 L/min
and a CPAP valve keeping the mPaw typically between 25 and 35 cm H_2O,[21] which
provides oxygenation to the patient. Ventilation is provided by a piston-driven vibrating
diaphragm. The rate of the diaphragm is set somewhere between 3 and 10 Hz.
The power set on the diaphragm determines the tidal volume of each breath
and is reflected in the oscillatory pressure amplitude (ΔP).

Typically, the settings on HFOV include the FIO_2, the mPaw, diaphragm Hz and ΔP.
Oxygenation is controlled through increasing the mPaw and FIO_2 if required. Ventilation is controlled through the ΔP and Hz. Contrary to initial beliefs, a decrease in Hz
actually improves ventilation by allowing a larger V_T. It cannot be predicted how
patients will respond to HFOV at various settings.

When initiating HFOV, patients are started with a setting of 100% FIO_2 and a mPaw
about 5 cm H_2O greater than that found on a conventional ventilator. Patients are
frequently recruited using recruitment maneuvers at the initiation of HFOV. If oxygenation does not improve, the mPaw is increased up to levels as high as 45 cm H_2O.
Once life-sustaining oxygenation has been achieved, the frequency and power are
adjusted to help minimize the amount of hypercarbia. If patients remain hypercarbic,
it is not uncommon to deflate the endotracheal tube cuff to improve ventilation. As the
patient improves, the FIO_2 is typically weaned to nontoxic levels (<50%) and then the
mPaw is gradually decreased. Conversion from HFOV to a conventional ventilator is
considered when mPaw is <25 cm H_2O.

For patients to tolerate HFOV, substantial sedation is required. Patients do not tend
to tolerate spontaneous respiration while on HFOV. If spontaneous breaths cannot be
extinguished using sedation alone, neuromuscular blockade is warranted. HFOV also
has marked effects on the cardiovascular system with potentially profound hypotension.[22,23] This is likely because the mPaw used tends to decrease preload profoundly;
however, attempts to treat preload with increased volume administration risks
reducing oxygenation. Judicious use of volume with the early administration of vasopressors seems reasonable in the management of these patients.

The overall effect of HFOV to date seems to be improved oxygenation. There are no
large-scale randomized trials showing improved survival with HFOV.[21] This is most
likely because of its use as a salvage strategy when conventional ventilation does
not provide adequate support. Data show that with the initiation of HFOV, the Pao_2/
FIO_2 ratio typically improves. In 1 multicenter trial, there was a nonsignificant trend
toward survival in the HFOV population compared with a conventional ventilation

arm.[24] The upcoming OSCILLATE trial which will be enrolling patients with early ARDS may provide greater insight into potential improved outcomes with HFOV.

Extracorporeal Membranous Oxygenation

Extracorporeal membranous oxygenation (ECMO) represents the final possible salvage modality in patients with severe respiratory failure. ECMO is the technique of providing long-term cardiopulmonary bypass support typically for days to weeks when conventional and/or unconventional ventilator modalities result in continuing hypoxia, profound hypercarbia, and/or hemodynamic compromise. ECMO is only a supportive therapy that provides time for other curative measures to act, including the body's natural immune system and time. In general survival for adult patients undergoing ECMO for respiratory support is between 40% and 70%.[25]

There are 2 primary forms of ECMO, venovenous (VV) and venoatrerial (VA). In VV ECMO, deoxygenated blood is extracted from the patient, oxygenated extracorporally, and returned to the patient's venous circulation close to the right atrium. This process results in a higher venous Po_2, which is then circulated through the lungs and then to the rest of the body using the patient's native cardiac function. VV ECMO is accomplished by either 2 single lumen catheters typically placed in the internal jugular and femoral veins or newer venovenous double lumen catheters (VVDL) placed in the internal jugular vein.

VA ECMO is designed to provide respiratory and cardiac support using catheters placed in the venous and arterial circulatory systems. Blood is withdrawn from the venous circulation, oxygenated, and returned to the patient's arterial circulation. Depending on the age and condition of the patient, a variety of methods for access to the patient's vasculature are available. In the adult, femoral venous and femoral arterial cannulation is preferred.

Randomized trials of adult ECMO are rare, similar to most high-technology/surgical therapies. During the original trial at 9 centers, 48 patients were managed using conventional ventilation and 42 patients received VA ECMO.[26] Survival in each group was 4 patients, which was not significantly different. Criticisms of the trial were: the technology that was implemented was immature, the centers involved were inexperienced, and the intervention of ECMO support occurred too late to affect survival.

In 2009, Peek and colleagues[27] published the results of the Conventional Ventilation or ECMO for Severe Adult Respiratory Failure (CESAR) trial. This trial randomized 180 patients with severe ARDS (Murray score >3 or pH <7.20) to care either at a tertiary care center or a single ECMO center. Of patients referred to the ECMO center 75% received ECMO therapy. Survival was 63% at 6 months for those patients referred to the ECMO center and 47% for those treated at tertiary care centers. Six of the patients in the ECMO group died in or pending transfer to the ECMO center. Criticisms of this trial include the lack of a standardized protocol for care at the tertiary care centers and a high rate to transfer mortality in the ECMO referral group.[28]

Historically, ECMO has been a limited resource. This has forced providers to seriously consider potential ECMO candidates long-term prognosis before the initiation of therapy. Each center has their own criteria for the initiation of ECMO; however, the requirement of anticoagulation and blood component transfusion for ECMO limits the patients who are eligible for therapy. Predictors of poor outcome for respiratory ECMO include advanced patient age, increased pre-ECMO ventilation duration, and diagnosis.[29] Absolute contraindications to ECMO include ongoing terminal disease that will not resolve or stabilize, inability to anticoagulate, intracranial hemorrhage, and refusal to receive blood products.

When the Patient with Respiratory Failure Requires a Surgical Procedure

Special preparations by the OR anesthesia and intensive care teams are required when the patient with severe respiratory failure on an advanced mode of ventilation needs a surgical procedure. It is imperative that communication regarding the patient's underlying condition and respiratory status occurs between the 2 teams. The ICU team should be responsible for optimizing the patient's oxygenation, ventilation, and hemodynamics before the patient goes to the OR.

Concerns for the OR anesthesia begin with how to safely transport the patient from the ICU to the OR. Most commonly, oxygenation and ventilation of an intubated ICU patient going to the OR occurs via resuscitation bag with high-flow oxygen and the addition of a PEEP valve. The patient in respiratory failure may not tolerate this mode of ventilation. If there is any question about the patient's safety for transport with a resuscitation bag, consider transporting the patient with an ICU ventilator. Newer models of ICU ventilators are lighter and easier to transport, provided enough personnel are available to assist. In the event an ICU travel ventilator is not available, every attempt should be made to bring the OR to the patient if possible, or consider an alternate technique for managing the situation. For example, a large intraabdominal fluid collection may be managed with percutaneous drainage rather than an exploratory laporotomy.

In addition, there is evidence that moving patients from the ICU is associated with an increased incidence of ventilator-associated pneumonia (VAP).[30,31] This increase in VAP rate may in part be caused by the patient being supine during transfer and transport, and patient movement causing shifting of respiratory secretions. Aggressive suctioning, using sterile in-line suction, checking for endotracheal tube cuff leaks, and maintaining the head of bed elevated may help to minimize this risk.

Once in the OR, the team must now focus on how to proceed with ventilation, oxygenation, the anesthetic plan, and management of hemodynamics. The patient in respiratory failure requiring an advanced mode of mechanical ventilation presents unique challenges to the anesthesia team. One of the main goals when providing care for such a patient should be to avoid additional lung injury leading to further deterioration in oxygenation. Careful attention should be paid to the preoperative PEEP settings and flow dynamics, and every effort should be made to replicate this environment in the OR. Most anesthesia machines in the OR, however, are not able to achieve the pressure limitations and flow characteristics of the ICU ventilators. In the case of the patient who may not tolerate ventilation with a conventional anesthesia machine, consider using the ICU ventilator in the OR.

If it is possible to use the anesthesia machine, the focus now shifts on how to best anesthetize this patient. Volatile agents are known to inhibit hypoxic pulmonary vasoconstriction.[32] Increasing intrapulmonary shunt will likely result in decreased oxygenation, which is not good in an already compromised patient. Conversely, experimental evidence has shown that inhalation agents (specifically sevoflurane) may actually be protective to injured lung by modulating the inflammatory response caused by activation of alveolar macrophages.[33] This concept is still theoretic. Until stronger evidence emerges, it remains most prudent to arrange for a total intravenous technique.

The effect of spontaneous ventilation on oxygenation during ventilation with APRV or BIPAP was discussed earlier. Surgical procedures requiring paralysis and abolition of spontaneous efforts may be detrimental. In this instance, the need for paralysis should be discussed with the surgical team, keeping in mind that the patient's best interests are paramount.

Hemodynamics as they relate to mechanical ventilation must also be considered. Positive-pressure ventilation and spontaneous ventilation during the respiratory cycle have significant effects on the patient's cardiovascular status. How the patient's hemodynamics react to alterations in airway pressures and the respiratory cycle must be monitored. These patients should have invasive monitors in place or placed intraoperatively to assist the anesthesiologist in assessing the patient's responses. Of utmost importance is the patient's intravascular volume status; it is highly recommended to avoid volume overload and favor hypovolemia in this population. It has been shown that in patients with ARDS fluid balance is directly correlated with mortality. Aggressive fluid resuscitation may worsen alveolar damage and inflammation.[34,35] Overall, the early implementation of vasopressors and/or inotropes seems prudent in this population in the OR. If the patient is receiving continuous renal replacement therapy (CRRT), and the procedure is expected to last more than 90 minutes, it would be prudent to continue to provide CRRT in the OR.

In the event a patient needs a surgical procedure on HFOV, it is imperative to fully discuss the entire procedure in detail with all providers involved. Frequently, these patients are not movable because of hypoxia or profound risk of technical complications during transport. For smaller procedures, it is reasonable to bring the OR to the patient, rather than risking moving the patient from the ICU. If the procedure is complex, requires specialized equipment, or has potentially high blood loss, it is then reasonable to move the patient from the ICU. If the patient is on HFOV, it is frequently possible to transport the patient using 100% Fio_2, high airway pressures, and inverse ratio ventilation. The goal should be to obtain an equivalent mPaw using a conventional ventilator to that provided on HFOV. This is usually not possible using the traditional low tidal volume strategies that have been proved to improve survival, and these settings are purely seen as salvage strategies. The acceptance of lower than normal Spo_2 as low as 80% with Pao_2 into the low 50s is also reasonable in these situations. Once in the OR, it is reasonable to resume treatment with HFOV during the procedure.

If a patient requires surgery while on ECMO, multiple provisions must be made by the anesthetic team. Bleeding and transport risks are the primary threat to the ECMO patient. Because of the high risk of bleeding, almost all surgical procedures should be completed in the OR. If a patient is on VV ECMO, it is reasonable to hold anticoagulation and attempt to normalize coagulation before surgery. This is because the risk from small venous emboli is very small relative to the risk of bleeding. VA ECMO patients are at a profound risk of stroke or other embolic events if they are not anticoagulated for prolonged periods of time. In the event a VA patient goes to the OR, a serious discussion of the risks and benefits of reducing anticoagulation must take place between all services. Regardless of the form of ECMO, there must be profound attention by the surgical service to achieving hemostasis during the procedure. The anesthesiologist should have all medications required for a cardiac bypass, including heparin and protamine. The anesthesiologist should have a firm understanding of the recommended ventilator settings that should be implemented in the event of ECMO circuit failure.

Despite the distinct challenges that patients with respiratory failure present to the anesthesiologist, a safe and smooth perioperative course can be achieved if the principles discussed in this article are followed.

REFERENCES

1. Torda TA. Alveolar-arterial oxygen tension difference: a critical look. Anaesth Intensive Care 1981;9(4):326–30.

2. Bernard GR, Artigas A, Brigham KL, et al. The American-European Consensus Conference on ARDS. Definitions, mechanisms, relevant outcomes, and clinical trial coordination. Am J Respir Crit Care Med 1994;149(3):818–24.
3. Ortiz RM, Cilley RE, Bartlett RH. Extracorporeal membrane oxygenation in pediatric respiratory failure. Pediatr Clin North Am 1987;34(1):39–46.
4. The Acute Respiratory Distress Syndrome Network. Ventilation with lower tidal volumes as compared with traditional tidal volumes for acute lung injury and the acute respiratory distress syndrome. The Acute Respiratory Distress Syndrome Network. N Engl J Med 2000;342(18):1301–8.
5. Slutsky AS. Lung injury caused by mechanical ventilation. Chest 1999; 116(Suppl 1):9S–15S.
6. Amato MB, Barbas CS, Medeiros DM, et al. Effect of a protective-ventilation strategy on mortality in the acute respiratory distress syndrome. N Engl J Med 1998;338(6):347–54.
7. Hess D, Kacmarek RM. Essentials of mechanical ventilation. 2nd edition. New York: McGraw-Hill; 2002. p. 382, xv.
8. Hess DR, Bigatello LM. The chest wall in acute lung injury/acute respiratory distress syndrome. Curr Opin Crit Care 2008;14(1):94–102.
9. Nichols D, Haranath S. Pressure control ventilation. Crit Care Clin 2007;23(2): 183–99, viii.
10. Marini JJ, Ravenscraft SA. Mean airway pressure: physiologic determinants and clinical importance–Part 2: clinical implications. Crit Care Med 1992;20(11):1604–16.
11. Marini JJ, Ravenscraft SA. Mean airway pressure: physiologic determinants and clinical importance–Part 1: physiologic determinants and measurements. Crit Care Med 1992;20(10):1461–72.
12. Rose L, Hawkins M. Airway pressure release ventilation and biphasic positive airway pressure: a systematic review of definitional criteria. Intensive Care Med 2008;34(10):1766–73.
13. Stock MC, Downs JB, Frolicher DA. Airway pressure release ventilation. Crit Care Med 1987;15(5):462–6.
14. Baum M, Benzer H, Putensen C, et al. [Biphasic positive airway pressure (BIPAP)– a new form of augmented ventilation]. Anaesthesist 1989;38(9):452–8 [in German].
15. Putensen C, Wrigge H. Clinical review: biphasic positive airway pressure and airway pressure release ventilation. Crit Care 2004;8(6):492–7.
16. Putensen C, Mutz NJ, Putensen-Himmer G, et al. Spontaneous breathing during ventilatory support improves ventilation-perfusion distributions in patients with acute respiratory distress syndrome. Am J Respir Crit Care Med 1999;159(4 Pt 1):1241–8.
17. Myers TR, MacIntyre NR. Respiratory controversies in the critical care setting. Does airway pressure release ventilation offer important new advantages in mechanical ventilator support? Respir Care 2007;52(4):452–8 [discussion: 458–60].
18. Burchardi H. New strategies in mechanical ventilation for acute lung injury. Eur Respir J 1996;9(5):1063–72.
19. Ferguson N, Stewart T. New therapies for adults with acute lung injury. High-frequency oscillatory ventilation. Crit Care Clin 2002;18(1):91–106.
20. Krishnan JA, Brower RG. High-frequency ventilation for acute lung injury and ARDS. Chest 2000;118(3):795–807.
21. Chan KP, Stewart T, Mehta S. High-frequency oscillatory ventilation for adult patients with ARDS. Chest 2007;131(6):1907–16.
22. Fort P, Farmer C, Westerman J, et al. High-frequency oscillatory ventilation for adult respiratory distress syndrome–a pilot study. Crit Care Med 1997;25(6): 937–47.

23. Bollen CW, van Well GT, Sherry T, et al. High frequency oscillatory ventilation compared with conventional mechanical ventilation in adult respiratory distress syndrome: a randomized controlled trial. Crit Care 2005;9(4):R430–9.
24. Derdak S, Mehta S, Stewart TE, et al. High-frequency oscillatory ventilation for acute respiratory distress syndrome in adults: a randomized, controlled trial. Am J Respir Crit Care Med 2002;166(6):801–8.
25. Brogan TV, Thiagarajan RR, Rycus PT, et al. Extracorporeal membrane oxygenation in adults with severe respiratory failure: a multi-center database. Intensive Care Med 2009;35:2105–14.
26. Zapol WM, Snider MT, Hill JD, et al. Extracorporeal membrane oxygenation in severe acute respiratory failure. A randomized prospective study. JAMA 1979; 242(20):2193–6.
27. Peek G, Mugford M, Tiruvoipati R, et al. Efficacy and economic assessment of conventional ventilatory support versus extracorporeal membrane oxygenation for severe adult respiratory failure (CESAR): a multicentre randomised controlled trial. Lancet 2009;374(9698):1351–63.
28. Zwischenberger J, Lynch J. Will CESAR answer the adult ECMO debate? Lancet 2009;374(9698):1307–8.
29. Hemmila M, Rowe S, Boules T, et al. Extracorporeal life support for severe acute respiratory distress syndrome in adults. Ann Surg 2004;240(4):595–605.
30. Bercault N, Wolf M, Runge I, et al. Intrahospital transport of critically ill ventilated patients: a risk factor for ventilator-associated pneumonia–a matched cohort study. Crit Care Med 2005;33(11):2471–8.
31. Kollef MH, Von Harz B, Prentice D, et al. Patient transport from intensive care increases the risk of developing ventilator-associated pneumonia. Chest 1997; 112(3):765–73.
32. Domino KB, Borowec L, Alexander CM, et al. Influence of isoflurane on hypoxic pulmonary vasoconstriction in dogs. Anesthesiology 1986;64(4):423–9.
33. Steurer M, Schlapfer M, Z'Graggen BR, et al. The volatile anaesthetic sevoflurane attenuates lipopolysaccharide-induced injury in alveolar macrophages. Clin Exp Immunol 2009;155(2):224–30.
34. Martin GS, Mangialardi RJ, Wheeler AP, et al. Albumin and furosemide therapy in hypoproteinemic patients with acute lung injury. Crit Care Med 2002;30(10): 2175–82.
35. Wiedemann HP, Wheeler AP, Bernard GR, et al. Comparison of two fluid-management strategies in acute lung injury. N Engl J Med 2006;354(24):2564–75.

Anesthetic Concerns in Patients Presenting with Renal Failure

Gebhard Wagener, MD[a], Tricia E. Brentjens, MD[a,b],*

KEYWORDS
- Renal function • Acute kidney injury
- Anesthesia • Renal failure

RENAL PHYSIOLOGY

The foremost function of the kidneys is to maintain fluid and electrolyte balance, by a tightly controlled system that is able to maintain homeostasis even in perilous metabolic situations. Other tasks include the excretion of metabolic waste products, control of vascular tone, and regulation of hematopoesis and bone metabolism.

The kidneys are the best-perfused organ per gram of tissue and receive 20% of the cardiac output. Global renal blood flow is autoregulated and is kept constant at a mean arterial pressure of 50 to 150 mm Hg in normotensive patients.[1] Blood flow to the glomerulus is regulated through the afferent and efferent sphincters, which adjust the glomerular filtration pressure. Depending on this filtration pressure a large amount of fluid (approximately 120 mL/min) is filtered into the capsular space of the Bowman capsule and then into the tubuli. Most of this glomerular filtrate is reabsorbed in the distal tubules of the inner medulla: active adenosine triphosphate (ATP) pumps move NaCl into the interstitium while water follows passively across an osmolar gradient. Urine and plasma osmolality are regulated by the feedback mechanism of the loop of Henle: increased interstitial NaCl concentrations (ie, as a result of hypovolemia) lead to an increased reabsorption of water and a decrease in urine output.

Renal blood flow is heterogenous. The renal cortex receives approximately 90% of renal blood flow, whereas the metabolically active renal medulla receives only about

---

[a] Division of Vascular Anesthesia and Division of Critical Care, Department of Anesthesiology, Columbia University, 630 West 168th Street, New York, NY 10032, USA
[b] Post Anesthesia Care Unit, New York Presbyterian Hospital, Presbyterian Campus, New York, NY, USA
* Corresponding author. Department of Anesthesiology, Columbia University, 630 West 168th Street, New York, NY 10032.
E-mail address: tb164@columbia.edu

Anesthesiology Clin 28 (2010) 39–54
doi:10.1016/j.anclin.2010.01.006
1932-2275/10/$ – see front matter © 2010 Elsevier Inc. All rights reserved.

anesthesiology.theclinics.com

10%. Tissue P_{O_2} is 50 to 100 mmHg in the cortex, whereas it can be as low as 10 to 15 mmHg in the medullary thick ascending limb. The renal medulla extracts 79% of delivered oxygen compared with only 18% in the renal cortex, which renders the renal medulla extraordinarily sensitive to ischemia.

In response to hypotension, systemic activation of the sympathetic and adrenal systems leads to redistribution of renal blood flow within the kidneys preferentially toward the metabolically active medulla and inner cortex.[2] Initially there is a preservation of glomerular filtration rate (GFR) and renal function, but with prolonged or more severe ischemia, active NaCl pumps in the thick ascending limb break down and sodium reabsorption decreases. Chemoreceptors in the macula densa of the juxtaglomerular apparatus detect the increased intraluminal chloride concentration and release renin. Renin then causes constriction of the afferent arteriole and a dramatic decrease of GFR that leads to a further reduction of urine output and oliguric renal failure ensues. Without the feedback mechanism of the macula densa, GFR would remain high (120 mL/min), water could not be reabsorbed, and fatal dehydration would occur within hours.[3]

The kidneys are able to tolerate substantial insults while maintaining adequate function despite this theoretic vulnerability to ischemia. Multiple and severe insults are required to cause an injury severe enough to manifest a clinically relevant decrease of renal function (**Fig. 1**). The most common cause of perioperative renal injury is ischemia-reperfusion injury. Ischemia-reperfusion injury causes tubular necrosis and apoptosis, especially of the medullary thick ascending loop of Henle. During reperfusion there is an influx of proinflammatory cells, neutrophils, and macrophages, which

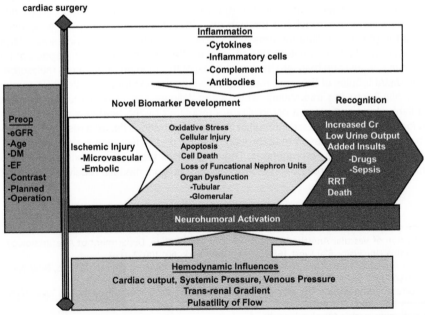

Fig. 1. Risk factors, mechanisms of injury and means of detection for AKI in relation to cardiac surgery. (*From* Bellomo R, Auriemma S, Fabbri A, et al. The pathophysiology of cardiac surgery-associated acute kidney injury (CSA-AKI). Int J Artif Organs 2008;31:167; with permission.)

release cytokines and radical oxygen species that further amplify necrosis and apoptosis.[4] In addition to direct injury, renal tubules become obstructed by cellular debris.[5]

Nephrotoxic insults caused by calcineurin inhibitors or aminoglycosides have a similar clinical presentation as ischemia-reperfusion injury even though the mechanism of injury is different. Calcineurin inhibitors cause profound afferent arteriolar vasoconstriction and decrease GFR,[6] whereas aminoglycosides cause tubular cell damage after reuptake into proximal tubular cells by megalin receptors.[7] Nonsteroidal antiinflammatory agents inhibit prostaglandin synthesis, which alone does not cause renal injury in normal subjects. In the setting of hypovolemia or in addition to other nephrotoxic insults, nonsteroidal antiinflammatory drugs may convert a small renal injury into overt renal failure as prostaglandin synthesis is essential to dilate the afferent arteriolar sphincter and maintain GFR.[8] Radiocontrast can cause renal injury, as it induces medullary vasoconstriction through activation of adenosin/endothelin receptors as well as by a direct cytotoxic effect of the high osmolality of radiocontrast.[9] The resultant clinical presentation is similar to ischemia-reperfusion injury, although usually a single insult with radiocontrast is not sufficient to induce clinically overt acute kidney injury (AKI).[10]

AKI

AKI often results from multiple insults and is frequently a consequence of a combination of prerenal azotemia and intrarenal acute tubular necrosis. In acute renal failure renal function deteriorates over hours or days. Primary renal diseases such as glomerulonephritis are rare in surgical populations and often associated with severe proteinuria and nephritic syndrome. Treatment of nephritic syndrome consists of replacement of protein loss and diuresis, steroids, and other immunosuppressive drugs that may reverse the symptoms.

Postrenal azotemia may be caused by renal calculi, tumors or even a blocked Foley catheter and rapid recovery of renal function will occur if the obstruction is removed or bypassed expeditiously. Iatrogenic injury of the ureter may occur during lower abdominal surgery, and the diagnosis of a dilated renal collecting system either by computed tomography scan or ultrasound should prompt rapid placement of either ureteral stents or nephrostomy tubes to relieve the pressure and avoid further, potentially irreversible injury to the kidney.

Reversible prerenal azotemia and acute tubular necrosis caused by medullary ischemia are two ends of a continuum. Prerenal azotemia is common and a physiologic response to hypovolemia. It increases tubular workload and decreases medullary blood supply. Any additional renal insult may result in sufficient medullary ischemia to cause acute renal failure. Urine output then decreases despite adequate intravascular filling, and waste products accumulate. The traditional division of prerenal versus intrarenal azotemia is therefore artificial, but may help guide treatment options, especially if further hydration may potentially reverse the condition. Once acute renal failure is established there is no intervention that has proven beneficial to expedite the recovery of renal function. In most cases renal function recovers spontaneously within days. However, it is essential to avoid further renal insults and support impaired physiologic systems to prevent progression to chronic renal failure (**Fig. 2**).

EPIDEMIOLOGY OF AKI

For many years the lack of a uniform definition and even a uniform term for renal injury has hampered clinical research of renal injury. The most commonly accepted term for

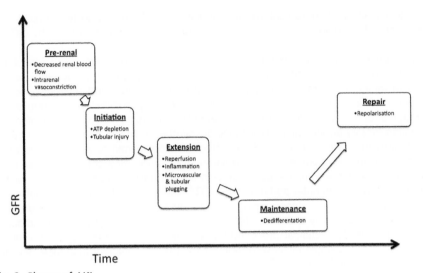

Fig. 2. Phases of AKI.

renal injury is acute kidney injury (AKI) as suggested by the American Society of Nephrology.[11] There is, however, no uniform definition of AKI. The Second International Consensus Conference of the Acute Dialysis Quality Initiative attempted to create a universally accepted definition of acute renal failure with the RIFLE criteria. The RIFLE criteria for AKI contain 5 categories (risk, injury, failure, loss, and end-stage kidney disease). The first 3 categories are defined by either percent change of serum creatinine or urine output criteria (**Fig. 3**).[12] The RIFLE criteria were initially widely recognized but later research showed that even small absolute changes of serum creatinine level affect morbidity and mortality.[13] The Acute Kidney Injury Network subsequently introduced a definition of AKI based on change of serum creatinine level of greater than 0.3 mg/dL within 48 hours after insult.[14]

Kheterpal and colleagues[15] recently reported that in a large national database 1% of all patients undergoing general surgery developed postoperative AKI. Patients developing AKI were more likely to be male, older, diabetic, and had more frequently a history of congestive heart failure, hypertension, ascites, or preoperative renal insufficiency. Emergency surgery doubled and intraperitoneal surgery more than tripled the risk for postoperative AKI. Patients who had AKI had a 3 times higher risk of postoperative morbidity and a fivefold increase in mortality.

AKI requiring renal replacement therapy (RRT) after cardiac surgery is rare (1%) but can be catastrophic and is associated with a mortality of greater than 60%. AKI based on the increase of serum creatinine level is more frequent but it is unclear if it is an independent contributor to mortality and morbidity or rather a reflection of more complex surgical procedures performed on complex medical patients.[16,17]

ASSESSMENT OF RENAL FUNCTION AND INJURY

Progress in renal protective strategies has been hampered by the lack of early sensitive markers of renal injury.[18] Direct measurements of GFR are cumbersome and rarely feasible. Substitute markers are required to estimate GFR but they have significant limitations.

GFR Criteria*   Urine Output Criteria

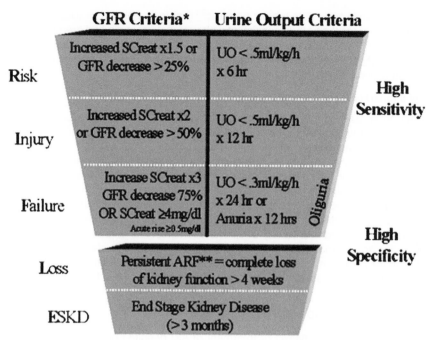

Fig. 3. Risk, injury, failure, loss of renal function, and end-stage kidney disease (RIFLE) criteria of AKI. (*From* Bellomo R, Ronco C, Kellum JA, et al. Acute renal failure – definition, outcome measures, animal models, fluid therapy and information technology needs: the Second International Consensus Conference of the Acute Dialysis Quality Initiative (ADQI) Group. Crit Care 2004;8:R206; with permission.)

Serum Creatinine

The most commonly used marker for renal function, serum creatinine level, is insensitive and slow to increase and, therefore, rarely detects renal injury rapidly enough for successful intervention. Small changes of serum creatinine level may represent large changes in GFR and there is not a linear relationship between creatinine and GFR. Serum creatinine requires time to accumulate and in the immediate perioperative period serum creatinine may even be decreased from preoperative levels because of dilution. Serum creatinine level is a marker of renal function and not injury.[19]

Urine Output

Urine output is not a reliable marker of renal function. Adequate urine output is usually associated with adequate renal function. Anuria is a sign of severe renal injury unless there is postrenal obstruction and requires immediate investigation. Low urine output may have various causes. Intra-abdominal surgery, especially laparoscopic, causes a decrease in renal blood flow and urine output that does not necessarily represent significant renal injury. Low urine output caused by hypovolemia may be secondary to easily reversible prerenal azotemia, which if left untreated can progress to acute renal injury.[20,21]

Fractional Excretion of Sodium

The fraction excretion of sodium (FeNa) measures the amount of filtered sodium that is excreted in the urine and is the most accurate test to aid the differential diagnosis of prerenal azotemia and acute tubular necrosis[22] (**Table 1**): FeNa % = $(U_{Na} \times P_{Cr})/(P_{Na} \times U_{Cr})$. A FeNa less than 1% is consistent with prerenal azotemia and greater than 2% with tubular injury. Concomitant use of diuretics decreases the diagnostic power of FeNa. Similarly, the fractional excretion of urea can be measured and may be a better reflection of renal function in patients receiving diuretics.[23]

Novel Biomarkers

Several novel biomarkers of renal injury and function have been studied in recent years, some of which have shown promising results. Serum cystatin C is a protein produced by all nucleated cells that is freely filtrated by the kidneys and not reabsorbed. Serum cystatin C is independent of age, muscle mass, sex, or race and reflects GFR better than serum creatinine.[24] Further studies are required to validate serum cystatin C as the better marker of renal function. Urinary neutrophil gelatinase-associated lipocalin is a protein produced by tubular cells as a response to injury. It is easily detected in the urine within minutes after experimental renal injury and has been studied in a variety of clinical scenarios.[25–28] It is highly sensitive and specific for acute renal injury and only slightly increased with chronic renal insufficiency. In the future it may be an ideal end point for studies evaluating renal protective strategies but more studies are required before its clinical use is feasible.[18,29]

RENAL PROTECTION AND TREATMENT OF AKI

There is no proven prophylaxis or treatment of AKI despite countless studies. Many interventions that were deemed successful in preclinical or early, small clinical trials were shown to be ineffective in larger studies that reflected realistic clinical scenarios.

Fluids

Maintaining renal blood flow and GFR through adequate hydration will prevent further renal injury and preserve renal function. Hydration has been shown to be effective in the prevention of contrast-induced nephropathy and other clinical scenarios of renal injury and is probably the best strategy to prevent progression to frank renal failure.[30]

Dopamine

Multiple large randomized trials and meta-analyses have found no therapeutic or prophylactic effect of dopamine on AKI.[31–33] Dopamine may increase urine output and may also be beneficial as treatment of low cardiac output states and treatment of bradycardia, leading to improved renal perfusion.

Bicarbonate

The alkalinization of urine with sodium bicarbonate is effective in the treatment of pigment-induced nephropathy such as rhabdomyolysis. It increases the solubility of

Table 1
Prerenal versus renal azotemia

Test	Prerenal	Renal
Urine osmolarity (mOsm/L)	<400	250–300
Urine creatinine/plasma creatinine ratio	>40	<20
Urine osmolarity/plasma osmolarity	>1.5	<1.0
Urine sodium concentration (mEq/L)	<20	>40
Fractional excretion of sodium (%)	<1	>1.1

myoglobin and therefore prevents formation of tubular precipitates.[34] Nephrotoxic free radicals are preferentially formed in acidotic environments, for example, through the Haber-Weiss reaction. Treatment with sodium bicarbonate decreases the formation of free radicals in contrast-induced nephropathy as well. A randomized trial found that pretreatment of bicarbonate reduced the incidence of contrast-induced nephropathy from 13.7% to 1.7%.[35]

Loop Diuretics/Mannitol

The rationale for using diuretics in the treatment of AKI is to flush out casts of necrotic cells that may obstruct renal tubuli. Loop diuretics also increase renal blood flow through increased prostaglandin synthesis and decrease metabolic workload of the tubuli by decreasing active sodium reabsorption. However, most clinical studies and a meta-analysis of randomized controlled trials found no effect of loop diuretics in the treatment or prevention of AKI.[36] Treatment with diuretics can lead to hypovolemia and further exacerbate renal hypoperfusion; therefore, it is imperative to ensure normovolemia before their use.

Acetyl Cysteine

Acetyl cysteine is a free radical oxygen scavenger and modulates nitric oxide synthesis after oxidative cell stress. Multiple studies had promising results and reported the efficacy of acetyl cysteine in the prevention of contrast-induced nephropathy when given early before the insult. Other studies were equivocal. Recent meta-analysis showed no effect in the prophylaxis of contrast-induced nephropathy[37] or in the prevention of AKI after major surgery.[38] Further studies with better-defined end points are necessary to obtain a better understanding of the clinical efficacy of acetyl cysteine.

EFFECT OF ANESTHESIA AND SURGERY ON RENAL FUNCTION

Clinical studies have failed to ascertain the benefit of one anesthetic technique over another in a general surgery population.[39] Care should be taken to maintain normovolemia and normotension to avoid decreases in renal perfusion. Volatile anesthetics in general cause a decrease in GFR likely caused by a decrease in renal perfusion pressure either by decreasing systemic vascular resistance (eg, isoflurane or sevoflurane) or cardiac output (eg, halothane). This decrease in GFR is exacerbated by hypovolemia and the release of catecholamines and antidiuretic hormone as a response to painful stimulation during surgery.[40] Recent studies have also found an amelioration of renal injury by volatile anesthetics, likely caused by a reduction in inflammation.[41]

Sevoflurane has been implicated as a cause of renal injury through fluoride toxicity. High intrarenal fluoride concentrations impair the concentrating ability of the kidney and may theoretically lead to nonoliguric renal failure. However, studies have failed to show a relevant effect in clinical practice. Sevoflurane is considered safe even in patients with renal impairment as long as prolonged low-flow anesthesia is avoided.[42,43]

Positive-pressure ventilation used during general anesthesia can decrease cardiac output, renal blood flow, and GFR. Decreased cardiac output leads to a release of catecholamines, rennin, and angiotensin II with the activation of the sympathoadrenal system and resultant decrease in renal blood flow. Insufflation of the abdomen during laparoscopic surgery has a similar effect on renal blood flow and GFR. The increased intra-abdominal pressure during laparoscopic surgery is transmitted directly to the kidneys and results in a further reduction of renal blood flow.[44]

The use of regional anesthesia techniques that achieve a sympathetic block of levels T4 to T10 may be beneficial to patients with kidney disease or those at high risk for postoperative AKI, as the sympathetic blockade attenuates catecholamine-induced renal vasoconstriction and suppresses cortisol and epinephrine release.[45] Epidural anesthesia has no effect on renal blood flow in healthy volunteers as long as normotension and isovolemia are maintained[46] and may reduce the incidence of postoperative AKI.[47]

Aortic cross-clamping or occlusion of the inferior vena cava during liver transplantation can cause renal injury that frequently progresses to AKI and substantially increases mortality and morbidity.[48–50] Cardiopulmonary bypass impairs renal blood flow and renal perfusion and may cause renal injury that might not be apparent early after surgery, as serum creatinine is often diluted in the early postoperative period.[51] Avoiding cardiopulmonary bypass with the use of off-pump coronary bypass grafting (CABG) does not necessarily reduce the degree of renal injury: hypotension, microemboli, and renal hypoperfusion during off-pump CABG may cause renal injury comparable to cardiopulmonary bypass,[52] and the results of clinical trials have been equivocal.

Avoiding intraoperative renal insults and maintaining isovolemia, adequate cardiac output, and renal perfusion pressure are the best interventions to prevent postoperative AKI and are more important than the choice of a specific anesthetic technique.

PHARMACOLOGIC MANAGEMENT OF THE PATIENT WITH RENAL FAILURE

Many drugs commonly used during anesthesia are dependent to some degree on renal excretion for elimination, and this must be taken into consideration when planning an anesthetic for a patient with renal dysfunction. Patients with renal disease are sensitive to barbiturates and benzodiazepines secondary to decreased protein binding. Some narcotic agents including morphine and meperidine should be used judiciously if at all as they have active metabolites and may have prolonged activity in the setting of renal dysfunction. Fentanyl and hydromorphone are better choices.[53,54] Succinylcholine can be used if the patient's serum potassium level is normal, but is best avoided if the potassium level is unknown. Cisatracurium and atracurium are nondepolarizing muscle relaxants that do not rely on renal function for their elimination, but are metabolized by ester hydrolysis and Hoffmann elimination. Neuromuscular reversal agents rely on renal excretion and, therefore, their effects will be prolonged.[55] Many antimicrobial agents must be dosed according to renal function. Nonsteroidal antiinflammatory agents should be avoided in renal insufficiency or AKI as they may exacerbate renal injury.

COMPLICATIONS OF RENAL FAILURE AND ITS IMPLICATION FOR THE ANESTHESIOLOGIST

Patients with renal failure undergoing surgery are at a substantial risk for increased morbidity and mortality. Patients with renal failure often have other comorbidities, including hypertension, diabetes, peripheral vascular disease, and cardiac disease. Renal failure has various consequences on homeostasis that are not only restricted to water and electrolyte abnormalities, but affect many organ systems, making intraoperative management of these patients especially challenging.

These patients can be hemodynamically labile during surgery and anesthesia. For minor procedures such as an inguinal hernia repair or an arteriovenous fistula, routine anesthetic monitors are probably sufficient. For major surgery, the anesthesiologist should probably place an arterial line to allow for continuous blood pressure monitoring to optimize patient care. Venous access can be challenging as well, as these patients often have vascular disease and have had a dialysis access procedure, which precludes the use of that arm for venous access. It is important to take your time and make sure that there is adequate venous access for the planned procedure. Central venous access to enable monitoring of central venous pressures may be beneficial to guide fluid management in patients who are oliguric or anuric during major surgery.

Patients with chronic renal failure undergoing elective surgery should receive dialysis treatment the day before planned surgery to optimize their electrolyte, metabolic, and volume status. It is appropriate to minimize intravenous fluid administration in this patient population for minor surgery. The importance of maintaining euvolemia during major surgery cannot be overstated to maintain adequate preload, thus avoiding hypotension and potential organ hypoperfusion.

Neurologic sequelae, including confusion, sedation, or obtundation, can result from uremic encephalopathy.[56] Intubation for airway protection may be necessary in extreme cases. Volume overload can to lead to pulmonary edema and hypoxia. Ventilatory support may be necessary until adequate fluid removal has been achieved with dialysis or diuresis. In addition, renal failure with a resultant metabolic acidosis may require hyperventilation as respiratory compensation that may not be sustainable in the spontaneously breathing patient. Mechanical ventilation may be required until the acidosis is corrected. Blood gas analysis at the point of care can alert the anesthesiologist to metabolic derangements and hypoxemia.

Anemia is frequent in patients with chronic renal failure and is caused in part by a decrease in erythropoietin production. Patients with renal dysfunction are at an increased risk for bleeding as they have altered platelet function and decreased levels of von Willebrand factor. Uremic coagulopathy is caused by impaired platelet aggregation and adhesiveness. Preoperative dialysis may be indicated if uremia is suspected. Alternatively, desmopressin, a vasopressin analog that releases von Willebrand factor and increases factor VII levels, can be administered preoperatively or intraoperatively to help correct uremic coagulopathy.[57]

Patients with renal failure can develop various metabolic derangements, including hyperkalemia, hypocalcemia, hyperphosphotemia, and metabolic acidosis. Frequent checking of arterial blood gases and electrolytes at the point of care, if possible, allows for early intervention and correction of derangements intraoperatively. Hyperkalemia results from the inability of the medullary tubuli to excrete potassium. If chronic it may be well tolerated but acute hyperkalemia warrants aggressive treatment. The anesthesiologist should be especially vigilant in monitoring the electrocardiogram for peaked T waves or a widening of the QRS complex. Hyperkalemia may worsen with the use of depolarizing muscle relaxants, ie, succinylcholine, and it should be avoided unless preoperative serum potassium levels are known.

Rapid transfusion of multiple units of packed red blood cells may increase potassium levels significantly. Metabolic acidosis, which often occurs in renal failure, worsens transfusion-induced hyperkalemia and may trigger arrhythmias and cardiac arrest.[58] The use of a cell saver device to prewash packed red blood cells or intraoperative continuous venovenous hemodialysis (CVVHD) should be considered in patients with restricted renal function who are likely to require many blood transfusions to prevent complications from hyperkalemia.

Treatment of hyperkalemia should be ideally aimed at the removal of excess potassium but temporizing interventions are warranted as well. Intravenous insulin moves extracellular potassium intracellularly by activating skeletal muscle Na-K ATP-dependent pumps. Usually 10 units of regular insulin intravenously are given together with

25 mL glucose 50% and glucose levels should be measured frequently afterwards. Intravenous calcium does not decrease plasma levels of potassium, but rather stabilizes the myocardium, preventing cardiac arrhythmias. Extravasation can cause severe skin necrosis and calcium should be given through a central venous catheter when possible. An increase in minute ventilation if the patient is mechanically ventilated results in an increase in plasma pH and a decrease in potassium levels. Treatment with sodium bicarbonate may increase plasma pH and drive potassium intracellularly; however, this effect is only a temporizing measure.

Treatment of hyperkalemia with loop diuretics increases potassium excretion. Cation exchangers such as sodium polystyrene sulfonate (Kayexalate) lowers potassium by binding intestinal potassium and excreting it in the stool. Sodium polystyrene sulfonate can be given orally or as a rectal enema. Treatment with sorbitol promotes osmotic diarrhea and amplifies the potassium-lowering effect but can lead to intestinal injury and colonic necrosis in patients with an ileus or after intestinal surgery and is not practical intraoperatively. If all of these interventions fail and hyperkalemia persists or becomes symptomatic, hemodialysis should be initiated as soon as possible.

Acidosis is common in acute renal failure and is often a result of the combination of impaired renal excretion of acid and an overproduction of lactic acid, for example secondary to septic shock. Hyperventilation of the mechanically ventilated patient helps to normalize pH but the spontaneously breathing patient is often unable to maintain an adequate minute ventilation to restore a normal pH. It is essential to recognize impending respiratory failure caused by increased breathing early and to intubate and mechanically ventilate the patient before cardiorespiratory collapse ensues. Severe metabolic acidosis at the end of surgery should preclude extubation until the metabolic derangements are corrected sufficiently to support spontaneous ventilation.[59]

Sodium bicarbonate is indicated in the mechanically ventilated patient when the pH decreases to less than 7.15.[60] At a pH of less than 7.15 most enzymatic and receptor-based systems fail to function properly (ie, catecholamine-based vasoconstriction). At this point treatment with sodium bicarbonate may restore the effectiveness of exogenous catecholamines and vascular tone. Sodium bicarbonate may also be indicated when bicarbonate loss and not an overproduction of acid is the cause for acidosis, as with the loss of bicarbonate through diarrhea or in renal tubular acidosis. Sodium bicarbonate should be given slowly to avoid overproduction of carbon dioxide. Carbon dioxide can easily traverse intracellularly, converting to carbonic acid and causing paradoxic intracellular acidosis.

Traditionally normal saline was the preferred intravenous fluid for patients with renal failure as it contains no potassium. However, recent studies reported that normal saline can cause a hyperchloremic metabolic acidosis that may increase the incidence of hyperkalemia more often than the use of a lactated Ringer solution (K 4 mEq/L).[61,62] The authors therefore recommend the use of lactated Ringer solution as the intravenous fluid in renal failure as long as hepatic function is sufficient to metabolize the lactate contained in the solution.

SPECIAL CONSIDERATIONS FOR PATIENTS WITH AKI

Perioperative renal failure is associated with a high morbidity and mortality. Preexisting renal insufficiency, advanced age, diabetes, and hypertension increase the risk of perioperative renal failure significantly. Assessment of the patient with acute renal failure presenting for surgery should include a thorough investigation of the cause. Subclinical sepsis may not be apparent except for an increase in serum creatinine level and white blood cell count but may unmask itself during anesthesia and surgery, causing vasodilatation and hemodynamic instability. Cardiogenic shock as a result of myocardial ischemia or cardiac tamponade may also present as acute renal failure. If the cause of the AKI is unclear further investigation is warranted before all surgery, except for emergencies.

Septic shock causes renal failure, resulting from a decrease in systemic vascular resistance and resultant hypotension, essentially causing a maldistribution of blood flow away from the kidneys and other vital organs that results in the reduction of trans-glomerular perfusion pressure and GFR. In addition, renal hypoperfusion causes direct medullary ischemia and acute tubular necrosis. Further injury occurs as sepsis induces leukocytic infiltration and apoptosis of the kidneys.[63] Fluid administration and the maintenance of adequate cardiac output are key to supportive treatment. In addition, treatment with vasopressors is often required to maintain adequate perfusion to vital organs by normalizing the systemic vascular resistance.

Cardiogenic shock results in hypoperfusion of the kidneys, decreased oxygen delivery, and acute tubular necrosis.[64] Decreased urine output and volume overload as a consequence of AKI may further worsen cardiogenic shock by increasing filling pressures beyond the plateau of the Frank-Starling curve, which can further exacerbate pulmonary edema and hypoxia. Reducing ventricular filling pressures with either diuresis or fluid removal via dialysis can improve cardiac output. If no significant improvement is achieved with the normalization of filling pressures, inotropic support or placement of an intra-aortic balloon pump may be required to maintain adequate coronary perfusion.

Nephrotoxic renal injury requires judicious fluid administration to maintain renal perfusion and prevent further insults. It is critical to avoid further renal injury caused by hypovolemia or hypoperfusion to avoid frank acute kidney failure requiring RRT.

Uremic pericarditis occurs in 5% to 20% of all cases of untreated renal failure and is caused by a hemorrhagic pericardial effusion as a consequence of uremic coagulopathy or serous effusions. Patients in acute renal failure complaining of pleuritic chest pain or presenting with a pericardial rub on physical examination should undergo echocardiograhy to confirm the diagnosis. Uremic pericarditis usually responds to treatment of the underlying uremia but pericardial drainage may be necessary in tamponade or hemodynamic compromise.[65]

Patients with AKI undergoing major surgery require invasive monitoring with at a minimum an arterial line to allow for continuous blood pressure monitoring and frequent blood draws to follow electrolytes and arterial blood gases closely. A central venous catheter to enable monitoring of central venous pressure may be useful in guiding fluid management if the patient is oliguric or anuric. A pulmonary artery catheter or transesophageal echocardiography aids in the assessment of cardiac function and volume status more closely and may be useful in patients presenting with septic or cardiogenic shock. The goal of the anesthesiologist in treating the patient with AKI intraoperatively is to optimize volume and hemodynamic status, thus maintaining renal perfusion and preventing further renal injury. Nephrotoxic agents should be avoided as well.

RRT

There are 5 indications for RRT: volume overload, hyperkalemia, severe metabolic acidosis, symptomatic uremia, and intoxication of dialyzable substances. Patients with end-stage kidney disease require RRT or a renal transplant. There are 2 basic modes of RRT in patients with end-stage kidney disease: intermittent hemodialysis and peritoneal dialysis. The patient with chronic renal failure on hemodialysis should undergo hemodialysis the day before elective surgery. If a patient with renal failure presents emergently for surgery and has an acute indication for dialysis but is hemodynamically unstable intraoperative continuous venovenous hemodialysis should be used if available.

The patient with acute renal failure who has not previously been dialyzed might require perioperative dialysis if any of the above indications are met. In addition, patients should undergo intraoperative dialysis if major blood loss with a large transfusion requirement is anticipated and the ensuing potassium load cannot be effectively managed through pharmacologic diuresis. Alternatively, cell saver can be used to wash packed red blood cells, effectively reducing the potassium load.

The mode of choice for intraoperative dialysis is continuous RRT unless the patient undergoes cardiopulmonary bypass and a dialysis membrane can be attached to the bypass circuit. Conventional hemodialysis is rarely feasible in the operating room as it may cause substantial hypotension. Any venovenous RRT requires the insertion of a large-bore, double-port venous catheter that allows flow rates of 150 to 300 mL/min.

Continuous RRT can be performed as either hemodialysis or hemofiltration. With continuous venovenous hemofiltration (CVVH) fluid is removed by creating a transmembrane pressure gradient. The amount of fluid removed depends on the blood flow and the surface area and water permeability of the filtration membrane. Solute removal is minimal and CVVH should be used intraoperatively only when volume overload is the sole indication for dialysis. During CVVHD solutes are removed by diffusion across a membrane against a concentration gradient, which allows for the effective removal of all dialyzable solutes and requires a blood flow rate of 150 to 300 mL/min and a dialysate flow rate of 2 to 6 L/min. Bicarbonate is preferable to acetate as a dialysate buffer as acetate can cause vasodilatation and hemodynamic instability.[66]

There is evidence that high-volume CVVHD is able to remove immunomodulatory substances such as tumor necrosis factors and endotoxins in septic shock that could decrease vasopressor requirements and improve outcome. Randomized controlled trials had conflicting results and further studies are required.[67,68]

SUMMARY

Patients presenting for surgery with renal insufficiency or failure present a significant challenge for the anesthesiologist. It is imperative that the anesthesiologist not only understands the management of these complex patients but also intervenes to prevent further renal injury during the perioperative period. Judicious fluid management, the maintenance of normovolemia, and avoidance of hypotension are priorities for the successful prevention of further renal injury. There may be instances when the use of CVVHD intraoperatively, if available, can be invaluable in the management of electrolyte and metabolic disturbances.

REFERENCES

1. Loutzenhiser R, Griffin K, Williamson G, et al. Renal autoregulation: new perspectives regarding the protective and regulatory roles of the underlying mechanisms. Am J Physiol Regul Integr Comp Physiol 2006;290:R1153–67.
2. Stein JH, Boonjarern S, Mauk RC, et al. Mechanism of the redistribution of renal cortical blood flow during hemorrhagic hypotension in the dog. J Clin Invest 1973;52:39–47.
3. Thurau K, Boylan JW. Acute renal success. The unexpected logic of oliguria in acute renal failure. Am J Med 1976;61:308–15.

4. Kinsey GR, Li L, Okusa MD. Inflammation in acute kidney injury. Nephron Exp Nephrol 2008;109:e102–7.
5. Bock HA. Pathogenesis of acute renal failure: new aspects. Nephron 1997;76: 130–42.
6. Shihab FS. Cyclosporine nephropathy: pathophysiology and clinical impact. Semin Nephrol 1996;16:536–47.
7. Nagai J, Tanaka H, Nakanishi N, et al. Role of megalin in renal handling of amino-glycosides. Am J Physiol Renal Physiol 2001;281:F337–44.
8. Harirforoosh S, Jamali F. Renal adverse effects of nonsteroidal anti-inflammatory drugs. Expert Opin Drug Saf 2009;8:669–81.
9. Itoh Y, Yano T, Sendo T, et al. Clinical and experimental evidence for prevention of acute renal failure induced by radiographic contrast media. J Pharmacol Sci 2005;97:473–88.
10. Weisbord SD, Mor MK, Resnick AL, et al. Incidence and outcomes of contrast-induced AKI following computed tomography. Clin J Am Soc Nephrol 2008;3: 1274–81.
11. Cerda J, Lameire N, Eggers P, et al. Epidemiology of acute kidney injury. Clin J Am Soc Nephrol 2008;3:881–6.
12. Bellomo R, Ronco C, Kellum JA, et al. Acute renal failure - definition, outcome measures, animal models, fluid therapy and information technology needs: the Second International Consensus Conference of the Acute Dialysis Quality Initiative (ADQI) Group. Crit Care 2004;8:R204–12.
13. Lassnigg A, Schmidlin D, Mouhieddine M, et al. Minimal changes of serum creatinine predict prognosis in patients after cardiothoracic surgery: a prospective cohort study. J Am Soc Nephrol 2004;15:1597–605.
14. Mehta RL, Kellum JA, Shah SV, et al. Acute Kidney Injury Network: report of an initiative to improve outcomes in acute kidney injury. Crit Care 2007;11:R31.
15. Kheterpal S, Tremper KK, Heung M, et al. Development and validation of an acute kidney injury risk index for patients undergoing general surgery: results from a national data set. Anesthesiology 2009;110:505–15.
16. Hoste EA, Cruz DN, Davenport A, et al. The epidemiology of cardiac surgery-associated acute kidney injury. Int J Artif Organs 2008;31:158–65.
17. Shaw A, Swaminathan M, Stafford-Smith M. Cardiac surgery-associated acute kidney injury: putting together the pieces of the puzzle. Nephron Physiol 2008; 109:p55–60.
18. Bonventre JV. Diagnosis of acute kidney injury: from classic parameters to new biomarkers. Contrib Nephrol 2007;156:213–9.
19. Soares AA, Eyff TF, Campani RB, et al. Glomerular filtration rate measurement and prediction equations. Clin Chem Lab Med 2009;47:1023–32.
20. Robert S, Zarowitz BJ. Is there a reliable index of glomerular filtration rate in critically ill patients? DICP 1991;25:169–78.
21. Bagshaw SM, Brophy PD, Cruz D, et al. Fluid balance as a biomarker: impact of fluid overload on outcome in critically ill patients with acute kidney injury. Crit Care 2008;12:169.
22. Pepin MN, Bouchard J, Legault L, et al. Diagnostic performance of fractional excretion of urea and fractional excretion of sodium in the evaluations of patients with acute kidney injury with or without diuretic treatment. Am J Kidney Dis 2007; 50:566–73.
23. Diskin CJ, Stokes TJ, Dansby LM, et al. The comparative benefits of the fractional excretion of urea and sodium in various azotemic oliguric states. Nephron Clin Pract 2009;114:c145–50.

24. Hojs R, Bevc S, Ekart R, et al. Serum cystatin C as an endogenous marker of renal function in patients with mild to moderate impairment of kidney function. Nephrol Dial Transplant 2006;21:1855–62.

25. Wagener G, Gubitosa G, Wang S, et al. Urinary neutrophil gelatinase-associated lipocalin and acute kidney injury after cardiac surgery. Am J Kidney Dis 2008;52: 425–33.

26. Wagener G, Gubitosa G, Wang S, et al. Increased incidence of acute kidney injury with aprotinin use during cardiac surgery detected with urinary NGAL. Am J Nephrol 2008;28:576–82.

27. Haase M, Bellomo R, Devarajan P, et al. Accuracy of neutrophil gelatinase-associated lipocalin (NGAL) in diagnosis and prognosis in acute kidney injury: a systematic review and meta-analysis. Am J Kidney Dis 2009;54:1012–24.

28. Wheeler DS, Devarajan P, Ma Q, et al. Serum neutrophil gelatinase-associated lipocalin (NGAL) as a marker of acute kidney injury in critically ill children with septic shock. Crit Care Med 2008;36:1297–303.

29. Coca SG, Yalavarthy R, Concato J, et al. Biomarkers for the diagnosis and risk stratification of acute kidney injury: a systematic review. Kidney Int 2008;73: 1008–16.

30. Trivedi HS, Moore H, Nasr S, et al. A randomized prospective trial to assess the role of saline hydration on the development of contrast nephrotoxicity. Nephron Clin Pract 2003;93:C29–34.

31. Bellomo R, Chapman M, Finfer S, et al. Low-dose dopamine in patients with early renal dysfunction: a placebo-controlled randomised trial. Australian and New Zealand Intensive Care Society (ANZICS) Clinical Trials Group. Lancet 2000; 356:2139–43.

32. Lassnigg A, Donner E, Grubhofer G, et al. Lack of renoprotective effects of dopamine and furosemide during cardiac surgery. J Am Soc Nephrol 2000;11:97–104.

33. Friedrich JO, Adhikari N, Herridge MS, et al. Meta-analysis: low-dose dopamine increases urine output but does not prevent renal dysfunction or death. Ann Intern Med 2005;142:510–24.

34. Better OS, Rubinstein I. Management of shock and acute renal failure in casualties suffering from the crush syndrome. Ren Fail 1997;19:647–53.

35. Merten GJ, Burgess WP, Gray LV, et al. Prevention of contrast-induced nephropathy with sodium bicarbonate: a randomized controlled trial. JAMA 2004;291:2328–34.

36. Ho KM, Sheridan DJ. Meta-analysis of frusemide to prevent or treat acute renal failure. BMJ 2006;333:420.

37. Kelly AM, Dwamena B, Cronin P, et al. Meta-analysis: effectiveness of drugs for preventing contrast-induced nephropathy. Ann Intern Med 2008;148:284–94.

38. Ho KM, Morgan DJ. Meta-analysis of N-acetylcysteine to prevent acute renal failure after major surgery. Am J Kidney Dis 2009;53:33–40.

39. Zacharias M, Conlon NP, Herbison GP, et al. Interventions for protecting renal function in the perioperative period. Cochrane Database Syst Rev 2008;(4): CD003590.

40. Kusudo K, Ishii K, Rahman M, et al. Blood flow-dependent changes in intrarenal nitric oxide levels during anesthesia with halothane or sevoflurane. Eur J Pharmacol 2004;498:267–73.

41. Lee HT, Ota-Setlik A, Fu Y, et al. Differential protective effects of volatile anesthetics against renal ischemia-reperfusion injury in vivo. Anesthesiology 2004; 101:1313–24.

42. Mazze RI. No evidence of sevoflurane-induced renal injury in volunteers. Anesth Analg 1998;87:230–1.

43. Gentz BA, Malan TP Jr. Renal toxicity with sevoflurane: a storm in a teacup? Drugs 2001;61:2155–62.
44. Annat G, Viale JP, Bui Xuan B, et al. Effect of PEEP ventilation on renal function, plasma renin, aldosterone, neurophysins and urinary ADH, and prostaglandins. Anesthesiology 1983;58:136–41.
45. Li Y, Zhu S, Yan M. Combined general/epidural anesthesia (ropivacaine 0.375%) versus general anesthesia for upper abdominal surgery. Anesth Analg 2008;106:1562–5.
46. Suleiman MY, Passannante AN, Onder RL, et al. Alteration of renal blood flow during epidural anesthesia in normal subjects. Anesth Analg 1997;84:1076–80.
47. Guay J. The benefits of adding epidural analgesia to general anesthesia: a meta-analysis. J Anesth 2006;20:335–40.
48. Rymarz A, Serwacki M, Rutkowski M, et al. Prevalence and predictors of acute renal injury in liver transplant recipients. Transplant Proc 2009;41:3123–5.
49. Barri YM, Sanchez EQ, Jennings LW, et al. Acute kidney injury following liver transplantation: definition and outcome. Liver Transpl 2009;15:475–83.
50. Cherr GS, Hansen KJ. Renal complications with aortic surgery. Semin Vasc Surg 2001;14:245–54.
51. Bellomo R, Auriemma S, Fabbri A, et al. The pathophysiology of cardiac surgery-associated acute kidney injury (CSA-AKI). Int J Artif Organs 2008;31:166–78.
52. Wagener G, Gubitosa G, Wang S, et al. A comparison of urinary neutrophil gelatinase-associated lipocalin in patients undergoing on- versus off-pump coronary artery bypass graft surgery. J Cardiothorac Vasc Anesth 2009;23:195–9.
53. Wagner BK, O'Hara DA. Pharmacokinetics and pharmacodynamics of sedatives and analgesics in the treatment of agitated critically ill patients. Clin Pharmacokinet 1997;33:426–53.
54. Liu LL, Gropper MA. Postoperative analgesia and sedation in the adult intensive care unit: a guide to drug selection. Drugs 2003;63:755–67.
55. Craig RG, Hunter JM. Neuromuscular blocking drugs and their antagonists in patients with organ disease. Anaesthesia 2009;64(Suppl 1):55–65.
56. Mahoney CA, Arieff AI. Uremic encephalopathies: clinical, biochemical, and experimental features. Am J Kidney Dis 1982;2:324–36.
57. Galbusera M, Remuzzi G, Boccardo P. Treatment of bleeding in dialysis patients. Semin Dial 2009;22:279–86.
58. Smith HM, Farrow SJ, Ackerman JD, et al. Cardiac arrests associated with hyperkalemia during red blood cell transfusion: a case series. Anesth Analg 2008;106:1062–9.
59. Elapavaluru S, Kellum JA. Why do patients die of acute kidney injury? Acta Clin Belg Suppl 2007;(2):326–31.
60. Dellinger RP, Levy MM, Carlet JM, et al. Surviving Sepsis Campaign: international guidelines for management of severe sepsis and septic shock: 2008. Crit Care Med 2008;36:296–327.
61. O'Malley CM, Frumento RJ, Hardy MA, et al. A randomized, double-blind comparison of lactated Ringer's solution and 0.9% NaCl during renal transplantation. Anesth Analg 2005;100:1518–24.
62. Khajavi MR, Etezadi F, Moharari RS, et al. Effects of normal saline vs lactated ringer's during renal transplantation. Ren Fail 2008;30:535–9.
63. Lerolle N, Nochy D, Guerot E, et al. Histopathology of septic shock induced acute kidney injury: apoptosis and leukocytic infiltration. Intensive Care Med 2010;36(3):471–8.
64. Ronco C, Haapio M, House AA, et al. Cardiorenal syndrome. J Am Coll Cardiol 2008;52:1527–39.

65. Gunukula SR, Spodick DH. Pericardial disease in renal patients. Semin Nephrol 2001;21:52–6.
66. Petroni KC, Cohen NH. Continuous renal replacement therapy: anesthetic implications. Anesth Analg 2002;94:1288–97.
67. Honore PM, Joannes-Boyau O, Gressens B. Blood and plasma treatments: the rationale of high-volume hemofiltration. Contrib Nephrol 2007;156:387–95.
68. McMaster P, Shann F. The use of extracorporeal techniques to remove humoral factors in sepsis. Pediatr Crit Care Med 2003;4(1):2–7.

The Anesthesia Patient with Acute Coronary Syndrome

Robert B. Schonberger, MD, MA, Ala S. Haddadin, MD, FCCP*

KEYWORDS

• Acute coronary syndrome • Antithrombin therapy
• Beta-blockade • Preoperative revascularization

Acute coronary syndrome (ACS), defined as unstable angina or myocardial infarction with or without ST-segment elevation,[1] is a common source of morbidity and mortality that presents unique management challenges for the anesthesiologist in the perioperative period. Coronary heart disease is the major pathology underlying ACS with a prevalence of approximately 16.8 million people in the United States.[2] In 2005, it is estimated that one in five deaths among United States adults was attributable to coronary heart disease.[2] Given such a widespread prevalence, every anesthesiologist will no doubt encounter patients with ACS and should know how to recognize and treat patients with this group of conditions.

Part I of this article will begin with a review of the current state of knowledge about the pathophysiology, diagnosis, and treatment of ACS outside of the perioperative period. Part II will focus on the perioperative period and highlights some aspects of particular relevance for the anesthesiologist caring for such patients. As part of this review of perioperative modalities for the management of patients suffering from ACS, the authors discuss the major guidelines and the evidence behind them and explore possible avenues for future research.

ACS encompasses three independent but related phenomena: (1) unstable angina, (2) myocardial infarction without ST-segment elevation (NSTEMI), and (3) myocardial infarction with ST-segment elevation (STEMI). While each of these entities is almost always a consequence of underlying coronary heart disease, the anesthesiologist should be aware of the important distinctions among them, particularly from the perspectives of treatment and outcome.

DIFFERENTIATING UNSTABLE ANGINA, NSTEMI, AND STEMI

Unstable angina should be distinguished from nonanginal chest pain syndromes, stable angina, and myocardial infarction. It is defined as myocardial ischemia of increasing duration or severity in the absence of cardiac myocyte necrosis.

Department of Anesthesiology, Yale University School of Medicine, 333 Cedar Street, TMP 3, PO Box 208051, New Haven, CT 06520-8051, USA
* Corresponding author.
E-mail address: ala.haddadin@yale.edu.

Anesthesiology Clin 28 (2010) 55–66
doi:10.1016/j.anclin.2010.01.001
1932-2275/10/$ – see front matter © 2010 Elsevier Inc. All rights reserved.

When evidence for myocardial necrosis is present in the form of positive blood creatinine phosphokinase—myocardial band or troponin levels, but is not accompanied by ST-segment elevation on an electrocardiogram, unstable angina has progressed to NSTEMI and is associated with a poorer outcome than is the case with biomarker-negative unstable angina. If there is evidence for ACS in the presence of ST-segment elevation of at least 1 mm in two adjacent leads, STEMI has occurred and is associated with the highest risk of poor outcome among the different degrees of ACS. Indeed, one-third of STEMI patients will be dead within 24 hours of the onset of ischemia.[3]

Diagnosis, Pathophysiology, and Treatment of ACS Outside the Perioperative Period

Diagnosis
In diagnosing ACS, a clinical history of worsening angina or anginal equivalents can be critical. Chest, jaw, shoulder, or upper abdominal discomfort may be presenting complaints—in addition to sweating, nausea, dyspnea and fatigue. Nevertheless, it is important to remember that as many as half of all myocardial infarctions remain clinically silent.[4] Therefore, in diagnosing ACS, the clinical history must be elicited in the context of risk factor recognition, physical examination, and, where appropriate, confirmatory laboratory studies. All patients with suspected ACS should receive an EKG and measurement of troponin blood levels for confirmation of diagnosis as well as risk stratification. Although these tests can confirm ACS, they cannot definitively rule it out. In the case of suspected ACS in which a nondiagnostic EKG and negative biomarker are found, a stress study that provokes ischemia may still lead to the diagnosis of unstable angina.[4] In contrast to the conscious patient, timely diagnosis of ACS in the patient undergoing a general anesthetic is obviously more difficult but can be facilitated by interpretation of the EKG, echocardiography, and changes in hemodynamics. Trends in filling pressures and cardiac output as seen on a pulmonary artery catheter can also be key in making a timely diagnosis.

Pathophysiology
Angina, as opposed to noncardiac chest pain, is a manifestation of cardiac ischemia and occurs when the oxygen supply of the myocardial tissue is insufficient relative to the demand. The supply–demand mismatch of angina can have many etiologies including impaired myocardial oxygen supply from anemia, hypoxia, atheroembolic events, microvascular impairment, or low perfusion pressures as well as increased myocardial oxygen demand from tachycardia, hypertrophy, and increased wall-stress.

Outside of the perioperative period, acute myocardial infarction is almost always a consequence of coronary artery thrombosis.[5] Such thrombosis most commonly occurs as a consequence of acute plaque rupture, although this has been shown to exhibit gender differences, with acute plaque rupture accounting for approximately 80% of coronary thrombosis in men versus 60% in women.[6]

Because of their critical role in coronary thrombosis, identification of plaques that are at high risk for rupture has been the object of much research. Plaques at the highest risk for acute rupture exhibit a thin fibrous cap overlying a necrotic, macrophage-rich core.[7] It is important to note that such plaques generally are found in places with less than 75% luminal stenosis, which may be the reason that revascularization in patients with chronic stable angina and preserved systolic function has not been shown to decrease the risk of subsequent myocardial infarction or death from coronary artery disease.[8] To understand this finding, one must remember that revascularization generally targets areas of the most severe coronary stenosis and, while treating such lesions may reduce anginal symptoms, it does nothing to reduce the risk of plaque rupture in areas with less critical stenosis.

Plaque erosion, as opposed to acute plaque rupture, is also a common pathophysiologic phenomenon leading to coronary blockage particularly in younger patients. It occurs in areas of a coronary artery where thrombus has come into direct contact with the coronary intima where the endothelial cell layer has been breeched. It is a morphology that is particularly common among smokers and young females presenting with coronary thrombosis and may highlight the importance of endothelial cell dysfunction to ACS. Finally, calcified nodules at the site of thrombosis is the third most common morphology underlying acute coronary blockage.[8]

The pathophysiology underlying the development and progression of coronary artery plaques is obviously varied, but the common risk factors first identified in the Framingham Heart Study and subsequently confirmed and modified in numerous studies include age, diabetes, smoking, family history, hypertension, and total and LDL cholesterol levels.[9] Elevated levels of high-sensitivity C-reactive protein (hs-crp), a systemic marker of inflammation, are also associated with increased risk. Therapy to improve any of the modifiable risk factors above is well demonstrated to reduce the risk of ACS.

Treatment

In order to effectively treat the patient who presents for surgery with ACS, it is critical for the anesthesiologist to bear in mind the several etiologies of myocardial ischemia while formulating a treatment plan. Maintenance of sufficient arterial oxygenation, coronary perfusion pressure, and hemoglobin concentration, as well as minimization of myocardial oxygen consumption, are always essential in cases of myocardial ischemia. However, identifying the priority of one particular factor over others may be paramount in particular clinical scenarios and may prevent the patient with unstable angina from progressing to myocardial infarction. Moreover, if infarction does occur, proper management can limit the size and hemodynamic impact of the infarcted tissue on the patient both in the perioperative period as well as in the long-term.

If the anesthesiologist is to understand the rationale behind perioperative management of acute coronary syndromes, it is critical to have an understanding of the standard of care outside of the operating room. With a solid understanding of the way the cardiologist approaches ACS, the anesthesiologist will be well-equipped to handle the same entity in the perioperative period. Accordingly, the present section reviews the treatment of ACS outside of the operating room.

Optimal treatment of patients with ACS remains a point of continued study and is generally stratified according to what type of ACS is occurring. Given the atheroembolic nature of the vast majority of ACS, there is a widespread consensus that patients presenting with ACS outside of the perioperative period should receive both antiplatelet and antithrombin therapy. Antiplatelet therapy is generally accomplished with aspirin or, where aspirin is contraindicated, an ADP-receptor antagonist such as clopidogrel.[4] Antithrombin therapy may include heparin, low-molecular weight heparin, or direct thrombin inhibitors. Part II addresses the need for the anesthesiologist to consider anticoagulant therapy within the surgical milieu but, outside of the operating room, it is considered a mainstay of treatment.

In all varieties of ACS, continuous monitoring for arrhythmia as well as treatment with oxygen, nitroglycerin, and analgesics are instituted unless contraindicated. While treatment with beta-blockade is considered a standard of care for long-term postmyocardial infarction treatment, recent evidence has highlighted the need to be wary of acute IV initiation of beta-blockade in patients with ACS because of the risk of worsening cardiogenic shock.[10] The complicated issue of the role of beta-blockade for primary prevention and treatment of ACS in the perioperative period is discussed in detail below.

Outside of the acute setting, statin therapy, which reduces cholesterol as well as high-sensitivity C-reactive protein, has been shown to be effective for primary prevention of major coronary events[11] as well as for reducing the risk of death and major cardiac events for patients following ACS.[12] Inhibition of the renin-angiotensin-aldosterone system, in addition to smoking cessation and other risk factor modification, are also staples of long-term treatment but play little if any role in the typical armamentarium of the anesthesiologist.

For patients suffering from STEMI, urgent attempts at reperfusion to minimize the extent of cardiac myocyte necrosis are the mainstay of treatment. Referral for primary percutaneous coronary intervention (PCI), depending on the availability of timely and skilled interventional cardiology, is the preferred reperfusion modality in STEMI. A great deal of evidence demonstrates that rapid initiation of PCI improves outcomes as compared with thrombolysis in these patients.[13] Nevertheless, where PCI is not available, thrombolytic therapy should be offered to appropriate patients suffering from STEMI. In the acute phase, placement of an intra-aortic balloon pump may be lifesaving until revascularization can occur.[14]

In contrast to STEMI, patients with unstable angina or NSTEMI are not generally triaged for emergent reperfusion therapy. In patients with ACS who are not having an STEMI, the present consensus points in favor of stratifying patients into lower and higher risk groups for whom optimization of medical management versus attempted early invasive revascularization are recommended, respectively. As discussed below, the decision to go to PCI for the patient who may need urgent surgery becomes more difficult given the need for acute anticoagulation and the recommendations for prolonged dual antiplatelet therapy following revascularization, particularly in the case of drug-eluting stents.

According to American College of Cardiology/American Heart Association (ACC/AHA) guidelines,[4] factors that would recommend toward an early invasive strategy outside of the perioperative period include:

1. Recurrent angina or ischemia at rest or with low-level activities despite intensive medical therapy
2. Elevated cardiac biomarkers (TnT or TnI)
3. New or presumably new ST-segment depression
4. Signs or symptoms of heart failure
5. New or worsening mitral regurgitation
6. High-risk findings from noninvasive testing
7. Hemodynamic instability
8. Sustained ventricular tachycardia
9. PCI within 6 months
10. Prior coronary artery bypass graft
11. High-risk score
12. Reduced left-ventricular function (ejection fraction <40%).[4]

These guidelines refer to the patient not scheduled for surgery. In the case of the perioperative situation, separate ACC/AHA guidelines make clear that for patients with high-risk unstable angina or NSTEMI, revascularization should be attempted before nonurgent, noncardiac surgery.[15]

A recent meta-analysis has suggested that the above guidelines may be particularly appropriate for women.[16] In one such study, the authors found that the benefit of an invasive strategy in terms of a reduced rate of death, myocardial infarction, or rehospitalization with ACS was significant and comparable for men and women if they had elevated cardiac biomarkers. However, in patients without elevated troponins, men still showed a trend toward improved risk with an invasive strategy, whereas women did not exhibit a trend toward any benefit.[16] Accordingly, conservative treatment of women with lower risk profiles along the lines of the ACC/AHA guidelines may be particularly advantageous.

Summary of ACS Outside the Perioperative Period

In sum, the acute treatment for ACS outside of the perioperative period depends on what type of ACS is occurring. The approach to all ACS should involve an attempt to identify and treat the underlying cause to prevent or minimize infarction. During that process it is critical to optimize the oxygen balance of the myocardium, limit coagulation and platelet function, monitor for arrhythmia, support hemodynamics as necessary, and rapidly determine the need for and timing of attempts at revascularization.

PART II: PERIOPERATIVE ACS
Epidemiology of ACS in the Perioperative Period

The estimated incidence of perioperative myocardial infarction depends on the population of patients and type of surgery being considered, as well as on the case definition and frequency of cardiac biomarker testing. For unselected patients over 40 years of age, a pooled incidence of 2.5% has been quoted in the literature.[17] On the other end of the scale, high-risk patients who were routinely screened for subclinical myocardial infarction had an incidence of postoperative troponin elevations as high as 25%.[17]

Clearly, a useful discussion of the incidence of ACS for prognostic purposes necessitates differentiating patients according to their risk profile. Accordingly, several attempts to model perioperative cardiac risk have been made, beginning with the Goldman criteria in 1977. In the Goldman and colleagues[18] paper, the nine independent cardiac risk factors included (1) the presence of a third heart sound or jugular venous distention; (2) recent myocardial infarction; (3) frequent premature ventricular contractions; (4) premature atrial contractions or rhythm other than sinus; (5) age over 70 years; (6) intraperitoneal, intrathoracic, or aortic operation; (7) aortic stenosis; (8) emergency operation; and (9) poor general medical condition.[18]

Over the years, other systems of risk assessment have been developed. The current ACC/AHA guidelines[15] follow the system described in 1999 by Lee and colleagues[19] who formulated the "Revised Cardiac Risk Index" using a population of patients greater than 50 years of age scheduled for nonurgent, noncardiac surgery. The index includes the following six risk factors: high-risk surgery, history of ischemic heart disease, history of congestive heart failure, history of cerebrovascular disease, preoperative treatment with insulin, and preoperative serum creatinine greater than 2.0 mg/dL. The validation cohort for this risk index demonstrated that the number of risk factors corresponded to the percentage of perioperative cardiac risk at the rate of zero risk factors at 0.4%, one to two at 0.9%, three at 7%, and more than three at 9%.

As the Lee and colleagues[19] study demonstrates, the greatest increase in risk (almost eightfold) occurs between the presence of two and three cardiac risk factors, and the ACC/AHA guidelines differentiate patients along this line as well.[15] Specifically, patients with poor functional capacity who are scheduled for intermediate or high-risk procedures are stratified into three groups depending on whether they have no risk factors, one to two risk factors, or three or more risk factors.

In addition, the Revised Cardiac Risk Index offers a sobering reminder to anesthesiologists who may harbor the illusion that they can avoid anesthetizing patients with active ACS. Even if one excludes caring for patients with known ACS who present for urgent surgery, any practitioner with a reasonable breadth of patients is bound to encounter situations in which he or she must treat a patient who has experienced a major cardiac event while under his or her care on the operating room table.

Perioperative Risk Modification

Whereas ACS on the operating room table will inevitably occur in the course of almost every anesthesiologist's career, several perioperative treatment modalities have been employed in the attempt to reduce the risk and impact of perioperative ACS.

Preoperative revascularization

The first possible modality for risk reduction is to delay surgery entirely until an acute cardiac issue has been optimized either through medical management or invasive revascularization. Following the ACC/AHA guidelines, any patient with recent or active myocardial infarction, decompensated congestive heart failure, uncontrolled arrhythmia, or a severe valvular lesion is classified as having an active cardiac condition and should undergo efforts to optimize his or her cardiac status (including medical management as well as possible cardiac surgery or percutaneous revascularization) before undergoing nonemergent noncardiac surgery.[15] In addition, patients who already have received an intracoronary stent should delay surgery until they have completed the minimum recommended course of dual antiplatelet therapy. For bare-metal stents, the interval should be at least 30 to 45 days and, for drug-eluting stents, one year.[17] However, it should be emphasized that the time guidelines for drug-eluting stents are but the latest iteration of a standard that has undergone repeated modification in the past decade as the risk of late and very late stent thrombosis has been further delineated.

Excluding the above patients, preoperative coronary revascularization and/or invasive evaluation are generally not indicated in patients with stable coronary artery disease unless such a procedure would be recommended independent of the patient's surgical status.[17] To understand the lack of benefit of preoperative revascularization, it is important to remember the major role of acute plaque rupture in ACS. While a patient with severe angina may benefit from the opening of a critically stenotic lesion that is the principal cause of the angina, patients with stable coronary disease are much more likely to suffer perioperative ACS because of acute plaque rupture rather than demand ischemia secondary to a discrete, stenotic lesion. As discussed above, acute plaque rupture generally occurs at sites without critical stenosis and unstable plaques can be present in patients with coronary lumina that appear normal on coronary angiography. Therefore, for patients with stable coronary disease, treatment efforts are better focused not on invasive revascularization, but rather on the stabilization of vulnerable plaques and the minimization of surgical stress on such plaques. An exception to this may be the patient with a high grade left main coronary artery stenosis in which the hemodynamic challenges of the operating room may carry a high risk of ischemia-induced myocardial compromise. In sum, coronary revascularization prior to noncardiac surgery is generally indicated only in unstable patients and in patients with particularly high-risk lesions of left main coronary artery.[20]

Perioperative medical management

For perioperative medical management, a variety of treatment modalities exist that may attenuate the cardiac risk of surgery. The use of beta-blockers and statins has been shown to attenuate cardiac risk in some patients. Aspirin is also generally continued perioperatively for most noncardiac surgeries. Other inhibitors of platelet function, such as ADP-receptor antagonists may also play a role in perioperative risk reduction. The maintenance of normothermia has been shown to reduce cardiac risk with the exception of situations in which therapeutic hypothermia may be used. Recent preliminary work has pointed to intensive perioperative insulin treatment for cardiac risk reduction, but this has yet to be replicated in additional studies. Ischemic preconditioning with volatile anesthetics may have a role as well.

Beta-blockade in the perioperative period is a topic of much study and increasing nuance. In high-risk patients, beta-blockade has been demonstrated in several studies to reduce the risk of perioperative myocardial infarction. However, caution is in order because administration of high-dose, day-of-surgery beta-blockade, in addition to reducing myocardial infarction, may increase the rate of all-cause mortality and stroke.[21] For the present article, rather than reviewing individual studies covering the perioperative use of beta-blockade, the authors recommend the relatively recent review article by Poldermans and colleagues[17] that offers both an insightful summary and a reasonably comprehensive list of references. That review as well as the most recent ACC/AHA update on the topic, recommend that patients on chronic beta-blocker therapy should continue them perioperatively, and patients with coronary artery disease may benefit from carefully titrated beta-blockade in the context of rigorous management of intraoperative hemodynamics.[17,22]

Statins have received much attention over recent years for their possible role in perioperative cardiac events via their so-called pleiotropic effects on plaque stabilization and attenuation of inflammation and their more well-known effects on levels of circulating low-density lipoproteins. A long acting statin (such as extended-release fluvastatin that has a biologic effect of at least 96 hours) is preferred preoperatively to best extend the anti-inflammatory effects into the postoperative period.[23] Statin therapy should be continued postoperatively, if possible, as there is a growing body of evidence that acute withdrawal increases markers of inflammation and oxidative stress and is associated with an increase in cardiac events.[17,24] The increasing consensus is that long-acting perioperative statins are both safe[25] and effective[26] for the reduction of perioperative cardiac events, particularly in high-risk patients.[17,22]

Antiplatelet therapy with aspirin must be carefully considered in consultation with both the surgeon and cardiologist but can generally be continued perioperatively for high-risk patients.[22] Exceptions to this are intracranial and possibly prostate surgery[22] as well as other situations such as the Jehovah's Witness patient in which surgical blood loss may carry a high risk of catastrophic outcome.

Recommendations for the ADP-receptor antagonist clopidogrel are somewhat idiosyncratic but, in general, studies suggest a significant increase in the risk of bleeding. Although the ACC/AHA recommendation is to stop it for five to seven days prior to elective coronary artery bypass surgery (CABG),[22] actual practice patterns depend on an individualized assessment of the risk of stopping anti-platelet agents. As mentioned above, the need for anti-platelet therapy is particularly important to consider in patients who have undergone stent placement during a percutaneous coronary intervention.

While intracoronary stent placement has improved PCI outcomes by reducing the rate of target vessel restenosis as compared to angioplasty alone,[27] it involves the introduction of a foreign body into the coronary artery that serves as a potential nidus for thrombosis. Drug-eluting stents were first approved in the United States in 2003, and they succeeded in further reducing the incidence of restenosis as compared with bare metal stents.[28] However, because they delay endothelialization, drug-eluting stents also prolong the period of time in which arterial thrombosis is likely to occur. Because arterial thrombosis is primarily a platelet-driven phenomenon, targeted anti-platelet regimens have become a mainstay of treatment for patients undergoing intracoronary stenting, and dual anti-platelet therapy with aspirin and an ADP-receptor antagonist is the current standard of care.[29,30] As mentioned above, dual anti-platelet therapy is recommended for a minimum of thirty days for bare metal stents and one year for drug-eluting stents. Any decision regarding adjustment of anti-platelet therapy perioperatively must consider carefully the relative risks of intraoperative bleeding and stent thrombosis and must be made in consultation with the surgeon and cardiologist. Important factors to consider in such situations include the patient's history, the type of stent, the time since stent implantation, the type of surgery, and the availability of timely PCI should it become necessary in the perioperative period. Patients at risk for stent thrombosis may be well-advised to consider arranging for surgery at a location that offers the option of emergent PCI should it become necessary.

Choices regarding anti-platelet therapy also may influence whether patients are offered a regional or neuraxial anesthetic technique. While aspirin and NSAIDS are not generally considered contraindications to regional anesthetics, clopidogrel is suspected to significantly increase the risk of spinal hematomas in neuraxial anesthesia.[31] Further complicating the choice of a regional anesthetic technique, practitioners should consider the possibility that they may find themselves managing a patient who requires emergent perioperative PCI in whom an epidural or regional catheter has already been placed.[32]

The newer antiplatelet ADP-receptor antagonist therapies ticagrelor[33] and cangrelor[34] appear promising in ACS with certain favorable pharmacologic features compared with clopidogrel. First, they give inhibition that is more complete and more rapid onset of action compared with clopidogrel. More importantly for the anesthesiologist, they are completely reversible, making their use attractive before knowledge of the coronary anatomy and for those who require noncardiac surgery with a stent already in place. Two recent trials comparing clopidogrel with cangrelor in patients undergoing PCI did not show superiority of cangrelor to clopidogrel in their primary endpoints,[34,35] but the secondary outcome of stent thrombosis was reduced with the use of cangrelor.[35] As newer and more reversible inhibitors of platelet function and coagulation become available in the coming years, the anesthesiologist's role as a perioperative manager of hemostasis will become increasingly important, especially in patients at high risk for ACS.

The use of a forced warm-air device for maintenance of intraoperative normothermia has also been shown to reduce the incidence of perioperative cardiac events.[36] The relevant study looked at patients with risk factors for coronary artery disease scheduled for thoracic, abdominal, or vascular surgeries. In this high-risk group, the number needed to treat was just over 20 patients. While this was only a single study, it was a randomized trial with robust results that has quickly led to increased awareness of the importance of perioperative normothermia. Indeed, Medicare quality improvement efforts now include perioperative normothermia in their pay-for-performance incentives.

The ideal temperature management for cardiac surgeries is beyond the scope of this article but must incorporate the need for hypothermic cerebral and cardiac protection during cardiopulmonary bypass.

A continuous insulin infusion as compared with intermittent insulin boluses was recently shown to reduce the combined incidence of all-cause mortality, heart failure, and myocardial infarction in vascular surgery patients.[37] Although the study was unblinded and from a single center, they enrolled over 200 subjects and demonstrated a number needed to treat of 11.4 patients. Given the risk and potentially catastrophic morbidity stemming from hypoglycemia, the introduction of continuous insulin infusions into the perioperative period must be done only in the context of a knowledgeable and astute anesthesia care team. It also remains unknown but of great interest to see how insulin infusions will impact patients scheduled for nonvascular surgery in which the cardiac risk is lower but the risk of hypoglycemia remains similar.

The use of volatile anesthetic agents in patients at high risk for cardiac events may be beneficial, presumably secondary to ischemic preconditioning effects, a post-conditioning effect, and also to an effect on apoptosis of the at-risk myocardium. Several human studies have shown a benefit to these agents in surrogate cardiac markers as compared with propofol or a balanced opioid technique in coronary artery bypass surgery patients.[22] Most of the available clinical data on the cardioprotective effects of volatile anesthetics to date are confined to coronary surgery patients. Cromheecke and colleagues demonstrated preserved cardiac function and improved cardiac biomarkers after aortic valve surgery when inhalation anesthetics were used intraoperatively as compared to a total intravenous technique,[38] however these findings run against the findings of Landoni and colleagues. Who found no benefit to the use of desflurane instead of propofol in mitral valve surgeries.[39]

Whether the suggestion of cardioprotection with inhalation anesthetics can be convincingly established in the cardiac operating room or extrapolated to noncardiac surgery remains to be seen. Furthermore, a mortality benefit in any population has yet to be demonstrated. Nevertheless, the role for and potential modalities of ischemic preconditioning will very likely be a fruitful source of research in the coming decade.

Intraoperative Management of Patients with ACS

Patients who develop a clinical picture worrisome for ACS intraoperatively require close consultation between the anesthesiology and surgical teams. Every effort should be made to reduce the patient's exposure to hemodynamic stressors beyond what is absolutely necessary and, if it is possible for surgery to be truncated or aborted, every consideration should be given to this option.

The anesthesiologist and surgeon should be aware of the treatment of ACS outside of the perioperative period and should treat the patient, insofar as possible, in accordance with those guidelines. A thorough understanding of the general approach to ACS will serve the anesthesiologist well intraoperatively. For example, a patient with prior coronary stenting who presents intraoperatively with hemodynamic instability and frank ST-elevation concerning for acute stent thrombosis should be scheduled, if possible, for emergent revascularization. With intraoperative ACS, just as outside of the operating room, the anesthesiologist should maximize myocardial oxygenation, minimize cardiac work, maintain hemodynamics, treat arrhythmias, and institute aspirin therapy as soon as the risk of surgical bleeding becomes acceptably low.

Cardiogenic shock is defined as low blood pressure unresponsive to fluids in the setting of elevated filling pressures, low cardiac output, and signs of tissue hypoperfusion. For patients in cardiogenic shock that is not rapidly corrected with pharmacologic support, the placement of an IABP is an ACC/AHA class I recommendation[13] (assuming that there is no significant aortic valve incompetence). Once an IABP is placed, it can remain as a lifesaving bridge before revascularization or placement of a more permanent ventricular assist device.

Opportunities for Future Research

Many issues remain unresolved in the perioperative treatment of ACS. Some of the major questions currently being investigated include (1) clarifying the proper population, dose, timing, and type of beta blockade that will be beneficial; (2) a better delineation of the role of perioperative statins; (3) the exploration of as yet undetermined preoperative treatment modalities for plaque stabilization and myocardial protection as well as for control of coagulation; (4) the development and identification of cardioprotective anesthetic strategies; and (5) the involvement of anesthesiologists in the long-term care of surgical patients through programs designed to identify patients with modifiable risk factors and refer them to the appropriate primary care setting.

Summary of ACS Within the Perioperative Period

The above brief review of ACS demonstrates why the patient with ACS should be considered among the patients "too sick for anesthesia." Induction of anesthesia and surgery introduce a patient into an environment prone to hypoxia, hypotension, hypertension, drops in hemoglobin, arrhythmogenic electrolyte abnormalities, increased inflammation, acute stress, and the need for avoidance of anticoagulation. It would be difficult to imagine a patient more ill suited for such a milieu than the patient suffering from an acute coronary syndrome.

REFERENCES

1. Gibbons RJ, Fuster V. Therapy for patients with acute coronary syndromes—new opportunities [comment]. N Engl J Med 2006;354(14):1524–7.
2. American Heart Association. Heart disease and stroke statistics—2009 Update. Dallas (TX): American Heart Association; 2009.
3. Antman EM, Anbe DT, Armstrong PW, et al. ACC/AHA guidelines for the management of patients with ST-elevation myocardial infarction: a report of the American College of Cardiology/American Heart Association Task Force on Practice Guidelines (Committee to Revise the 1999 Guidelines for the Management of Patients with Acute Myocardial Infarction). Circulation 2004;110(9):e82–292 [Erratum appears in Circulation 2005;111(15):2013–4].
4. Anderson JL, Adams CD, Antman EM, et al. ACC/AHA 2007 guidelines for the management of patients with unstable angina/non ST-elevation myocardial infarction: a report of the American College of Cardiology/American Heart Association Task Force on Practice Guidelines (Writing Committee to Revise the 2002 guidelines for the management of patients with unstable angina/non ST-elevation myocardial infarction): developed in collaboration with the American College of Emergency Physicians, the Society for Cardiovascular Angiography and Interventions, and the Society of Thoracic Surgeons: endorsed by the American Association of Cardiovascular and Pulmonary Rehabilitation and the Society for Academic Emergency Medicine. Circulation 2007;116(7):e148–304 [Erratum appears in Circulation 2008;117(9):e180].
5. Davies MJ, Woolf N, Robertson WB. Pathology of acute myocardial infarction with particular reference to occlusive coronary thrombi. Br Heart J 1976;38(7):659–64.
6. Falk E. Pathogenesis of atherosclerosis. J Am Coll Cardiol 2006;47(Suppl 8):C7–12.
7. Virmani R, Burke AP, Farb A, et al. Pathology of the vulnerable plaque. J Am Coll Cardiol 2006;47(Suppl 8):C13–8.
8. Aguiar-Souto P, Silva-Melchor L, Ortigosa-Aso FJ. Chronic stable angina [comment]. N Engl J Med 2005;353(14):1524 [author reply].
9. Wilson PW, D'Agostino RB, Levy D, et al. Prediction of coronary heart disease using risk factor categories. Circulation 1998;97(18):1837–47.
10. Antman EM, Hand M, Armstrong PW, et al. 2007 focused update of the ACC/AHA 2004 guidelines for the management of patients with ST-elevation myocardial

infarction: a report of the American College of Cardiology/American Heart Association Task Force on practice guidelines: developed in collaboration with the Canadian Cardiovascular Society endorsed by the American Academy of Family Physicians: 2007 Writing group to review new evidence and update the ACC/AHA 2004 guidelines for the management of patients with ST-elevation myocardial infarction, writing on behalf of the 2004 Writing Committee. Circulation 2008; 117(2):296–329 [Erratum appears in Circulation 2008;117(6):e162].

11. Ridker PM, Danielson E, Fonseca FAH, et al. Rosuvastatin to prevent vascular events in men and women with elevated C-reactive protein [comment]. N Engl J Med 2008;359(21):2195–207.

12. Cannon CP, Braunwald E, McCabe CH, et al. Intensive versus moderate lipid lowering with statins after acute coronary syndromes [comment]. N Engl J Med 2004;350(15):1495–504 [Erratum appears in N Engl J Med 2006;354(7):778].

13. Keeley EC, Boura JA, Grines CL. Primary angioplasty versus intravenous thrombolytic therapy for acute myocardial infarction: a quantitative review of 23 randomised trials [comment]. Lancet 2003;361(9351):13–20.

14. Antman EM, Anbe DT, Armstrong PW, et al. ACC/AHA guidelines for the management of patients with ST-elevation myocardial infarction—executive summary. A report of the American College of Cardiology/American Heart Association Task Force on Practice Guidelines (Writing Committee to revise the 1999 guidelines for the management of patients with acute myocardial infarction) [comment]. J Am Coll Cardiol 2004;44(3):671–719 [Erratum appears in J Am Coll Cardiol 2005;45(8):1376].

15. Fleisher LA, Beckman JA, Brown KA, et al. ACC/AHA 2007 guidelines on perioperative cardiovascular evaluation and care for noncardiac surgery: a report of the American College of Cardiology/American Heart Association Task Force on Practice Guidelines (Writing Committee to Revise the 2002 Guidelines on Perioperative Cardiovascular Evaluation for Noncardiac Surgery): developed in collaboration with the American Society of Echocardiography, American Society of Nuclear Cardiology, Heart Rhythm Society, Society of Cardiovascular Anesthesiologists, Society for Cardiovascular Angiography and Interventions, Society for Vascular Medicine and Biology, and Society for Vascular Surgery. Circulation 2007;116(17):e418–99 [Erratum appears in Circulation 2008;118(9):e143–4].

16. O'Donoghue M, Boden WE, Braunwald E, et al. Early invasive vs conservative treatment strategies in women and men with unstable angina and non–ST-segment elevation myocardial infarction: a meta-analysis [comment]. JAMA 2008;300(1):71–80.

17. Poldermans D, Hoeks SE, Feringa HH. Pre-operative risk assessment and risk reduction before surgery. J Am Coll Cardiol 2008;51(20):1913–24.

18. Goldman L, Caldera DL, Nussbaum SR, et al. Multifactorial index of cardiac risk in noncardiac surgical procedures. N Engl J Med 1977;297(16):845–50.

19. Lee TH, Marcantonio ER, Mangione CM, et al. Derivation and prospective validation of a simple index for prediction of cardiac risk of major noncardiac surgery. Circulation 1999;100(10):1043–9.

20. Garcia S, Moritz TE, Ward HB, et al. Usefulness of revascularization of patients with multivessel coronary artery disease before elective vascular surgery for abdominal aortic and peripheral occlusive disease. Am J Cardiol 2008;102(7): 809–13.

21. Group PS, Devereaux PJ, Yang H, et al. Effects of extended-release metoprolol succinate in patients undergoing non-cardiac surgery (POISE trial): a randomised controlled trial [comment]. Lancet 2008;371(9627):1839–47.

22. Fleischmann KE, Beckman JA, Buller CE, et al. 2009 ACCF/AHA focused update on perioperative beta blockade incorporated into the ACC/AHA 2007 guidelines on perioperative cardiovascular evaluation and care for noncardiac surgery. J Am Coll Cardiol 2009;54(22). DOI:10-1026/j.jacc.2009.07.010.

23. Schouten O, Hoeks SE, Welten GMJM, et al. Effect of statin withdrawal on frequency of cardiac events after vascular surgery. Am J Cardiol 2007;100(2):316–20.

24. Heeschen C, Hamm CW, Laufs U, et al. Withdrawal of statins increases event rates in patients with acute coronary syndromes [comment]. Circulation 2002; 105(12):1446–52.

25. Schouten O, Kertai MD, Bax JJ, et al. Safety of perioperative statin use in high-risk patients undergoing major vascular surgery. Am J Cardiol 2005;95(5):658–60.

26. Durazzo AES, Machado FS, Ikeoka DT, et al. Reduction in cardiovascular events after vascular surgery with atorvastatin: a randomized trial [comment]. J Vasc Surg 2004;39(5):967–75 [discussion: 75–6].

27. Fischman DL, Leon MB, Baim DS, et al. A randomized comparison of coronary-stent placement and balloon angioplasty in the treatment of coronary artery disease. Stent Restenosis Study Investigators. N Engl J Med 1994;331(8):496–501.

28. Sousa JE, Costa MA, Sousa AGMR, et al. Two-year angiographic and intravascular ultrasound follow-up after implantation of sirolimus-eluting stents in human coronary arteries. Circulation 2003;107(3):381–3.

29. Leon MB, Baim DS, Popma JJ, et al. A clinical trial comparing three antithrombotic-drug regimens after coronary-artery stenting. Stent Anticoagulation Restenosis Study Investigators. N Engl J Med 1998;339(23):1665–71.

30. Schomig A, Neumann FJ, Kastrati A, et al. A randomized comparison of antiplatelet and anticoagulant therapy after the placement of coronary-artery stents. N Engl J Med 1996;334(17):1084–9.

31. Horlocker TT, Wedel DJ, Benzon H, et al. Regional anesthesia in the anticoagulated patient: defining the risks (the second ASRA Consensus Conference on Neuraxial Anesthesia and Anticoagulation). Reg Anesth Pain Med 2003;28(3):172–97.

32. Popescu WM, Gusberg RJ, Barash PG. Epidural catheters and drug-eluting stents: a challenging relationship. J Cardiothorac Vasc Anesth 2007;21(5):701–3.

33. James S, Akerblom A, Cannon CP, et al. Comparison of ticagrelor, the first reversible oral P2Y(12) receptor antagonist, with clopidogrel in patients with acute coronary syndromes: rationale, design, and baseline characteristics of the PLATelet inhibition and patient Outcomes (PLATO) trial. Am Heart J 2009;157(4):599–605.

34. Harrington RA, Stone GW, Mcnulty S, et al. Platelet inhibition with cangrelor in patients undergoing PCI. N Engl J Med 2009;361(24):2318–29.

35. Bhatt DL, Lincoff AM, Gibson M, et al. Intravenous platelet blockade with cangrelor during PCI. N Engl J Med 2009;361(24):2330–41.

36. Frank SM, Fleisher LA, Breslow MJ, et al. Perioperative maintenance of normothermia reduces the incidence of morbid cardiac events [comment]. A randomized clinical trial. JAMA 1997;277(14):1127–34.

37. Subramaniam B, Panzica PJ, Novack V, et al. Continuous perioperative insulin infusion decreases major cardiovascular events in patients undergoing vascular surgery: a prospective, randomized trial [comment]. Anesthesiology 2009;110(5): 970–7.

38. Cromheecke S, Pepermans V, Hendrickx E, et al. Cardioprotective properties of sevoflurane in patients undergoing aortic valve replacement with cardiopulmonary bypass. Anesth Analg 2006;103(2):289–96.

39. Landoni G, Calabro MG, Marchetti C, et al. Desflurane versus propofol in patients undergoing mitral valve surgery. J Cardiothorac Vasc Anesth 2007;21(5):672–7.

Anesthetic Considerations for Patients with Advanced Valvular Heart Disease Undergoing Noncardiac Surgery

Jonathan Frogel, MD*, Dragos Galusca, MD

KEYWORDS

- Aortic stenosis • Aortic insufficiency • Mitral stenosis
- Mitral insufficiency • Valvular heart disease
- Noncardiac surgery

The prevalence of advanced valvular heart disease in the United States currently stands at 2.5% and is expected to increase considerably with the aging of the population.[1] With this anticipated increase in prevalence, anesthesiologists can expect to encounter an increasing number of patients with advanced valvular heart disease presenting for noncardiac surgery. Valvular heart disease has been recognized as a risk factor for perioperative cardiac morbidity for more than 30 years.[2] Although much attention has been paid to the perioperative implications and management of patients with preexisting coronary artery disease presenting for noncardiac surgery, similar literature regarding valvular heart disease is sparse. For example, the revised 2007 American College of Cardiology/American Heart Association (ACC/AHA) Guidelines on Perioperative Cardiovascular Evaluation and Care for Noncardiac Surgery consider severe aortic and mitral stenosis "active cardiac conditions" and recommend evaluation and treatment (ie, percutaneous valvuloplasty for mitral stenosis) before proceeding with elective surgery.[3] However, guidelines for the management of patients with severe valvular disease who require emergency surgery or are not candidates for valve repair/replacement are limited. This article reviews the anesthetic

Department of Anesthesiology, Henry Ford Hospital, 2799 West Grand Boulevard, Detroit, MI 48202, USA
* Corresponding author.
E-mail address: jfrogel1@hfhs.org

Anesthesiology Clin 28 (2010) 67–85
doi:10.1016/j.anclin.2010.01.008
1932-2275/10/$ – see front matter © 2010 Published by Elsevier Inc.

anesthesiology.theclinics.com

implications of symptomatic valvular heart disease and the management of patients with advanced cardiac valvular lesions presenting for noncardiac surgery.

AORTIC STENOSIS
Epidemiology

Aortic stenosis (AS) has long been considered an important risk factor for perioperative cardiac events. In patients undergoing noncardiac surgery, severe AS is correctly regarded as the most significant valvular lesion because of the complexity of its intraoperative management and the increased risk of adverse perioperative outcomes with which it has been associated. AS has a high prevalence in elderly people, and it has been associated with increased risk for perioperative morbidity and increased incidence of sudden death.[2,4,5] In 1977, Goldman showed that AS was one of the independent variables that increases the risk of perioperative myocardial infarction, ventricular tachycardia, and cardiac death.[2] A multifactorial clinical risk index was later proposed; critical/symptomatic AS was assigned the highest predictive value for perioperative cardiac events.[6] Later data showed that little increased morbidity occurred in patients with severe AS undergoing noncardiac surgery, suggesting that the institution of aggressive intraoperative monitoring and correction of hemodynamic instability likely play an important role in improving outcomes.[7]

Cause

The causes of AS can be roughly divided into congenital and acquired. In the adult population, the most commonly encountered congenital cause is bicuspid aortic valve (AV), accounting for more than 50% of cases of congenital AS.[8] The most frequently encountered causes of acquired AS are senile calcific degeneration, rheumatic heart disease, and infective endocarditis.[9,10] Senile calcification of the trileaflet AV is frequently present after the age of 70 years, and in many cases is diagnosed incidentally.[4] In an echocardiographic study, critical AS (valve area <0.8 cm^2) had a prevalence of 2.9% in elderly patients between 75 and 86 years of age.[11]

Symptoms

AS typically develops over decades, with an indolent course in many patients. Syncope, angina, and heart failure represent the classic symptom triad of severe AS (valve area <1 cm^2) and are associated with projected lifespan after onset of 5, 3, and 2 years, respectively. However, although clinical symptoms are highly predictive of significant disease, the absence of symptoms does not preclude the presence of severe stenosis. As compensatory mechanisms fail and symptoms occur, long-term prognosis worsens. For example, average survival without corrective surgery is less than 2 years following an episode of heart failure in patients with AS.[5]

Pathophysiology

The normal AV has an area of 2 to 4 cm^2 with severe AS currently defined by the following parameters: valve area less than 1 cm^2, mean transvalvular pressure gradient more than 40 mm Hg, and peak blood velocity more than 4 m/s.[12,13] In most cases of AS gradual narrowing of the valve orifice results in chronic obstruction to left ventricular flow and left ventricular pressure overload. In response to this pressure overload, concentric left ventricle hypertrophy (LVH) typically develops and normalizes the concomitant increase in wall tension seen secondary to the valvular stenosis. Contractility is usually preserved, maintaining a normal ejection fraction until late in the disease process.[14]

Although concentric hypertrophy helps preserve LV systolic function, it has delete-rious physiologic effects also. Because of increased ventricular mass and wall tension, myocardial oxygen demand increases significantly. In addition, capillary density is often inadequate in the hypertrophied ventricle,[8,15] leading to supply/demand mismatch and an increased risk of myocardial ischemia, even in the absence of coro-nary artery disease. Blood supply may be further compromised when coronary perfu-sion pressure (CPP) is reduced by either a reduction in aortic diastolic pressure or an increase in ventricular filling pressure. Underlying coronary artery disease can further aggravate this supply/demand mismatch.

Impairment of diastolic relaxation occurs secondary to concentric LVH (**Fig. 1**),[16] leading to increased isovolemic relaxation times and impeding early LV filling. Subop-timal relaxation necessitates higher left atrial pressures to drive early diastolic filling and to maintain adequate LV preload. In addition, impaired early diastolic filling makes the ventricle more dependent on the atrial contribution to maintain adequate preload. In fact, atrial systole may account for up to 40% of ventricular filling in patients with severe AS.

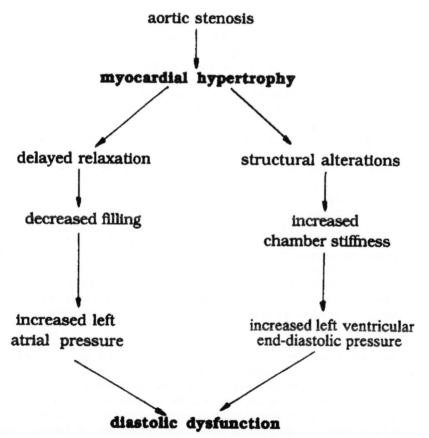

Fig. 1. Progression of concentric LVH and diastolic dysfunction in patients with AS. (*From* Hess OM, Villari B, Krayenbuehl HB. Diastolic dysfunction in aortic stenosis. Circulation 1993;87(Suppl 5):74; with permission.)

Anesthetic Considerations

In deciding to proceed with elective noncardiac surgery in patients with AS clinicians need to consider the feasibility of further medical optimization or suitability of the patient for preoperative intervention such as AV replacement or valvuloplasty. The decision needs to be tailored to each individual patient and clinical scenario. Comprehensive reviews of the preoperative clearance considerations for patients with AS can be found elsewhere. This section focuses on the anesthetic management of patients for whom the decision to proceed with surgery has already been made.

The pathophysiology of AS and its compensatory LVH dictate careful manipulation of hemodynamics in the perioperative period. The main goals are to maintain sinus rhythm, a relatively slow heart rate (HR), adequate intraventricular volume (preload), and systemic vascular resistance (SVR; afterload). Specifically, the increased myocardial oxygen demand and paucity of capillary blood supply seen in advanced disease make maintenance of adequate afterload and aortic diastolic pressure a necessity to minimize the risk of myocardial ischemia. By the same token, a slower HR, which decreases myocardial oxygen demand and increases coronary perfusion time, can prevent supply/demand ischemia in these patients. Maintenance of adequate afterload has an additional beneficial effect of driving preload, maintaining left atrial pressure and adequate left ventricular diastolic filling. Similarly, slower HRs help optimize left ventricular filling by maximizing diastolic time. In addition, carefully maintaining intravascular volume helps ensure adequate preload.

In patients with severe AS undergoing noncardiac surgery, the outcomes are related to a thorough preoperative evaluation and an appropriate perioperative anesthetic plan.[17] According to recently updated guidelines, patients with significant AS do not require preoperative antibiotics for the prevention of infective endocarditis unless there is a prior history of endocarditis.[18] Further anesthetic premedication should be tailored to the specific patient and should be carefully titrated. In general, anticholinergics should be used cautiously as they cause dose-dependent increases in HR. The decision to provide preoperative sedation and anxiolysis must balance the risks of oversedation and hypotension versus undersedation and increased sympathetic tone. Careful titration of preoperative sedation to avoid either extreme is crucial.

Anesthetic management should target the previously outlined hemodynamic goals and is especially crucial when a sympathetic response is expected such as during laryngoscopy, surgical stimulation, or emergence. Tachycardia should be avoided as it decreases diastolic filling time and cardiac output (CO), and can lead to severe hemodynamic compromise. In addition, the reduction of diastolic coronary perfusion and increase in myocardial oxygen demand observed during episodes of tachycardia can precipitate ischemia, life-threatening arrhythmias, and ultimately cardiac arrest. Thus, a defibrillator should be readily available in the operating room, and placed on the patient before positioning and sterile draping.[15] Severe bradycardia (HR <40 beats per minute) has to be prevented as it too can result in decreased CO and hypotension caused by the relatively fixed flow across the stenotic valve. This point is especially important in elderly patients in whom sinus node disease and reduced sympathetic responses may predispose to significant bradycardia. Ideally, HR should be kept in the range of 60 to 70 beats per minute. In mixed lesions, in which AS coexists with aortic insufficiency (AI), a higher HR may be better tolerated. Preservation of normal sinus rhythm is of great importance as atrial systole is necessary for maximizing LV preload. In the event of new-onset supraventricular arrhythmias with hemodynamic instability, prompt cardioversion should be used.

Patients with AS are preload dependent and appropriate intravascular volume must be assured before induction. Hypovolemia and vasodilation should be avoided and treated promptly should they occur. Special considerations apply when neuraxial anesthesia is chosen because of the undesirable decrease in SVR seen with sympathectomy. Continuous invasive arterial blood pressure monitoring and available vaso-constrictive therapy are advisable if neuraxial techniques are to be used.[15] An epidural technique may be preferable as it allows for incremental dosing and the avoidance of sudden changes in SVR. Alternatively, other regional techniques such as combined spinal-epidural anesthesia and continuous spinal anesthesia have been described with acceptable outcomes.[19,20]

If careful monitoring is assured, general anesthesia can offer excellent hemodynamic control. Certain medications such as opioids, midazolam, etomidate, and cis-atracurium may represent good choices, as they offer a relatively stable hemodynamic profile, and should be titrated to effect. Other medications, such as glycopyrolate, ketamine, and pancuronium may induce undesirable tachycardia. Propofol may decrease contractility and preload, and consequently, may worsen hemodynamic status. Thiopental may decrease contractility and preload, and is probably best avoided. Regardless of the anesthetic technique, all anesthetics should be titrated carefully to maintain SVR and CO throughout the procedure. Hypotension must be identified promptly and aggressively treated with an α agonist to assure adequate CPP and ventricular preload. Pure α agonists are the agents of choice because they do not cause tachycardia, and thus maintain adequate diastolic filling time.

Intraoperative monitoring should follow the recommendations of the American Society of Anesthesiologists (ASA). Electrocardiographic monitoring should include leads II and V5, although ischemia may be difficult to detect because of the presence of LVH and strain. As mentioned earlier, patients with AS can experience major decreases in CO and blood pressure with even minor changes in HR, preload, and afterload. It is therefore prudent to institute invasive arterial blood pressure monitoring before the induction of anesthesia. Central venous catheters offer the advantage of access to the central circulation for venous pressure monitoring and administration of pressors and inotropes as needed. The role of the pulmonary artery catheter (PAC) remains controversial as the evidence supporting improved outcomes with its use is absent, but it may be useful for carefully titrating volume status in the hands of practitioners experienced in placement and interpretation of data.[16] If PAC monitoring is used, wedge pressure can underestimate preload because of decreased ventricular compliance. Transesophageal echocardiography (TEE) offers the advantage of continuously monitoring preload, contractility, and regional wall motion changes but requires special expertise for image acquisition and interpretation. According to current ACC/AHA guidelines, surgical procedures with significant risk for myocardial ischemia and hemodynamic compromise are class IIa indications for intraoperative TEE monitoring.[21]

In conclusion, the anesthetic management of patients with AS should be tailored to the individual patient and is predicated on the maintenance of hemodynamic parameters within narrow ranges. Postoperative management should be considered a continuation of the intraoperative care and should focus on tight maintenance of preload, contractility, SVR, and CO. Strong consideration should be given to admitting AS patients to an intensive care unit for immediate postoperative care to ensure that these goals are met.

AI

Epidemiology

The incidence of AI in the general population is approximately 10%, with most cases in the trace/mild range of severity. The incidence of moderate/severe AI is less than 0.5%. Risk factors associated with AI on multiple logistic regression analysis are male gender and age.[22]

Cause

The cause of AI can be either congenital or acquired with changes affecting either the valve leaflets directly or the aortic root, thereby indirectly preventing normal leaflet coaptation.[23] Common acquired causes of leaflet dysfunction are infective endocarditis and rheumatic fever; bicuspid AV is the most widely encountered congenital cause of leaflet malfunction. Aortic root dilatation may be associated with collagen vascular disease, connective tissue disorders (ie, Marfan syndrome), aging, or chronic systemic hypertension.[24] AI may present with an acute or chronic onset. Chronic AI is more commonly encountered in patients undergoing noncardiac surgery. Acute AI may be associated with infective endocarditis, type A aortic dissection, or trauma, and represents a true surgical emergency.

Symptoms

Acute AI can be life threatening and can manifest with acute chest pain, dyspnea, and symptoms of cardiogenic shock. Chronic AI is usually asymptomatic, but progression of the disease may manifest with dyspnea, exercise-induced angina, tachycardia, and palpitations.

Pathophysiology

AI in its acute and chronic forms results in LV volume overload secondary to regurgitation of stroke volume from the aorta into the LV during diastole. In acute AI the sudden increase in regurgitant volume and ventricular preload and wall tension occurs in the absence of left ventricular compensatory mechanisms. This increase results in the dramatic presentation seen in this setting, including chest pain secondary to subendocardial ischemia, pulmonary edema secondary to the acutely increased LV diastolic pressure impeding normal diastolic filling, and organ dysfunction secondary to cardiogenic shock. In chronic AI the insidious course of the disease allows for compensatory mechanisms to come into play. Specifically, left ventricular dilatation occurs to accommodate increases in preload, and nonconcentric LVH develops to compensate for increased wall tension and stress. Myocardial oxygen supply/demand balance can usually be maintained for a longer period in chronic AI. Eventually, however, preload reserve is lost, and increases in afterload secondary to increased stroke volume cause increases in wall stress and decreased ejection fraction and the onset of overt symptoms (**Fig. 2**).[21]

Anesthetic Considerations

The anticipated surgical procedure, the patient's baseline functional status, and severity of disease all play important roles in the risk assessment and preoperative therapy for patients with AI. Acute AI almost always requires urgent cardiac surgical intervention and does not represent the focus of this review. Asymptomatic mild chronic AI is usually well tolerated and likely poses little additional perioperative patient risk. Patients with severe or symptomatic chronic AI should be considered for evaluation and medical optimization before elective surgery.[3]

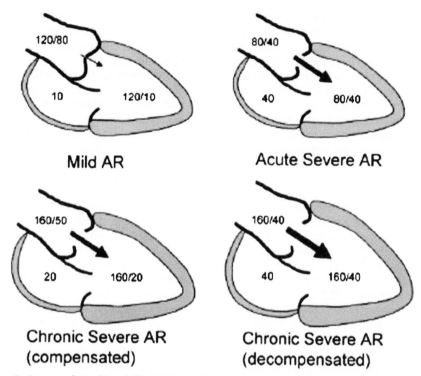

120/80	80/40
10 120/10	40 80/40
Mild AR	**Acute Severe AR**
160/50	160/40
20 160/20	40 160/40
Chronic Severe AR (compensated)	**Chronic Severe AR (decompensated)**

Fig. 2. Stages of AI. (*Top left*) Mild AI with preserved ventricular function and normal ventricular size. (*Top right*) Severe acute AI with normal left ventricular and atrial size, equalization of aortic and ventricular diastolic pressures, and severely increased left atrial pressures. (*Bottom left*) Compensated chronic severe AI with ventricular hypertrophy and mild dilatation of the LV. Systolic blood pressure and pulse pressure are increased and LV systolic function is maintained by a combination of hypertrophy and increased ventricular preload. (*Bottom right*) Decompensated chronic severe AI with a severely dilated and hypertrophied LV. Ventricular systolic function is typically impaired because of increased afterload, and diastolic function is decreased secondary to fibrosis and hypertrophy, leading to equalization of aortic and ventricular pressures and increase of atrial pressure. (*Modified from* Berkeredjian R, Grayburn PA. Valvular heart disease: aortic regurgitation. Circulation 2005;112:127; with permission.)

Hemodynamic management in patients with more severe forms of AI is focused on decreasing regurgitant volume and maximizing effective forward flow and CO. To this end, maintaining a relatively fast HR decreases time spent in diastole and, by extension, regurgitant volume. Similarly, afterload reduction decreases the aortic/ventricular gradient and can minimize regurgitant flow. In patients with AI secondary to aortic root disease (aneurismal dilatation), the risk of acute rupture dictates taking measures to ensure that ventricular ejection velocity and aortic wall stress are well controlled (usually through the use of β-blockers and avoidance of dramatic increases in sympathetic tone).

Current guidelines do not recommend prophylactic antibiotics to prevent infective endocarditis in patients with AI undergoing dental or surgical procedures, except in patients with history of prior endocarditis.[17] Maintenance of preoperative antihypertensive medications is likely beneficial in helping to maintain perioperative afterload reduction. In patients with significant aortic root disease, medications that help control aortic wall stress (β-blockers) should be continued also. Preoperative sedation/anxiolysis is not contraindicated in patients with AI because modest decreases in afterload are considered beneficial. Similarly, treatment with anticholinergics is not contraindicated because increases in HR may decrease regurgitant flow.

The anesthetic technique should be chosen with the aim of achieving the hemodynamic goals outlined earlier. General, neuraxial, and regional techniques can all be used safely. Regardless of the technique selected, avoiding sudden decreases in HR, increases in SVR, and myocardial depression is crucial.[23]

Hemodynamic monitoring decisions should be tailored to each clinical scenario. Minor surgical interventions do not usually require invasive monitoring. Patients with severe or symptomatic AI may benefit from invasive arterial blood pressure monitoring before induction of anesthesia. Central venous catheter placement should be considered for patients undergoing major surgery with anticipated intravascular volume shifts or blood loss and may facilitate fluid resuscitation and administration of vasodilators, should afterload reduction become necessary. In patients with severe AI and decompensated congestive heart failure, placement of a PAC may be prudent to allow for CO and SVR monitoring and to guide hemodynamic and fluid management. However, in severe AI, pulmonary capillary occlusion pressure may overestimate preload because of premature closure of mitral valve secondary to early increases in diastolic pressure.[15] TEE can be used to detect early myocardial depression.

Induction of general anesthesia can be safely achieved with agents such as propofol or thiopental. Ketamine may increase afterload and impede forward flow and should be used cautiously. Nondepolarizing muscle relaxants are all considered safe, with pancuronium offering the potential added benefit of HR increase. If succinylcholine is to be used episodes of bradycardia should be treated with anticholinergics. Special care should be taken during laryngoscopy, intubation, and other periods of stimulation to minimize increases in afterload. Maintenance of anesthesia with volatile agents, neuromuscular blockers, and opioids is acceptable, provided there is minimal myocardial depression. In advanced disease, LV dysfunction may require contractility augmentation with an inotrope such as dobutamine.

Postoperatively, special consideration should be given to patients with severe or symptomatic disease and to those who required aggressive intraoperative fluid resuscitation. These patients may be prone to the development of postoperative pulmonary edema as the effects of the anesthetic dissipate and afterload increases. Admission to the intensive care unit in the immediate postoperative period should be considered to guarantee tight hemodynamic control.

MITRAL STENOSIS
Epidemiology

Although the incidence of mitral stenosis has decreased dramatically in the United States, it is still a commonly encountered disease in the developing world, where the prevalence of rheumatic fever remains high. For example, in India the incidence of rheumatic fever is 6:1000 (compared with 0.5:1000 in developed countries), with nearly one-third showing symptoms of rheumatic heart disease and mitral stenosis.[25] In developed countries, the prevalence of mitral stenosis detected echocardiographically from all causes is 0.02% to 0.2%.[1]

Cause

Rheumatic heart disease is the most common cause of mitral stenosis. Susceptible patients may develop chronic inflammatory injury to the mitral valve following episodes of *Streptococcal A* infection. This chronic inflammation leads to progressive thickening and scarring of valvular and subvalvular tissue, ultimately causing clinically apparent mitral stenosis.[26] Other causes of acquired mitral stenosis include degenerative disease, mitral annular calcification with leaflet encroachment (particularly in elderly patients or those dependent on hemodialysis), systemic inflammatory diseases (eg, rheumatoid arthritis and systemic lupus erythematosus), endocarditis, carcinoid heart disease, and iatrogenic stenosis (ie, following mitral valvuloplasty).[27] Congenital mitral stenosis typically presents at an early age and is not addressed in this review.

Pathophysiology

The mitral valve orifice area normally measures 4 to 6 cm^2, allowing diastolic flow across the valve to occur with a minimal pressure gradient between the left atrium and LV. Overt symptoms of mitral stenosis (dyspnea, palpitations, syncope) are usually not apparent until the valve area is reduced to less than 1.5 cm^2. As mitral stenosis progresses and the valve orifice area decreases, left ventricular diastolic filling is impaired, requiring increased left atrial pressure to overcome the stenotic valve and maintain adequate left ventricular preload. Increased left atrial pressure results in left atrial enlargement, predisposing patients to supraventricular arrhythmias. Decreased atrial flow velocities place patients at risk for the development of intra-atrial thrombus formation and systemic embolization (**Fig. 3**).[28] The high left atrial pressures are transmitted back to the pulmonary venous and arterial circulation, resulting in increased lung water and pulmonary hypertension. Although this increase in pulmonary pressure may be completely reversible early in the course of the disease,

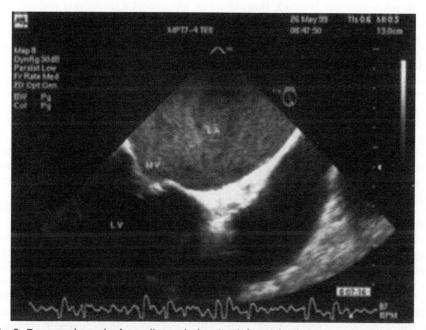

Fig. 3. Transesophageal echocardiograph showing left atrial enlargement and spontaneous echo contrast in a patient with mitral stenosis and atrial fibrillation. (*From* Vincelj J, Sokol I, Jaksic O. Prevalence and clinical significance of left atrial spontaneous echo contrast detected by transesophageal echocardiography. Echocardiography 2002;19:321; with permission.)

patients with long-standing mitral stenosis typically develop permanent changes to the pulmonary vasculature, resulting in an irreversible component of pulmonary hypertension. As the disease progresses, the ability of the right ventricle to function in the setting of increased pulmonary vascular resistance is impaired and signs and symptoms of right heart failure may predominate. Left ventricular systolic function is usually well preserved in patients with mitral stenosis.[29]

Anesthetic Considerations

Patients with symptomatic mitral stenosis should be carefully evaluated and optimized before noncardiac surgery whenever possible. Ideally, candidates for mitral valve reconstruction, replacement, or percutaneous valvuloplasty should have these procedures performed before proceeding with elective surgery.[3] This article focuses on the perioperative management of patients with mitral stenosis who are not candidates for the procedures outlined earlier or those who are presenting for emergency surgery.

Perioperative hemodynamic goals in patients with symptomatic mitral stenosis are predicated on maintaining adequate left ventricular diastolic filling and optimizing right heart function. The stenotic mitral valve acts as an impediment to diastolic filling. This impediment must be overcome to maintain adequate left ventricular stroke volume and CO. The stenotic valve leads to significantly impaired early diastolic filling, placing increased importance on atrial contraction (and by extension, sinus rhythm) to maintain left ventricular preload. Atrial fibrillation is often the precipitating event leading to the onset of dyspnea and definitive diagnosis.[22] Nearly half of all patients with symptomatic mitral stenosis develop chronic atrial fibrillation.[30] However, if sinus rhythm is present, it should be aggressively maintained as loss of the atrial kick can dramatically impair left ventricular preload. Regardless of the patient's underlying rhythm, HR should be well controlled as slower rates increase diastolic filling time and improve ventricular filling. Conversely, acute increases in HR can lead to dramatic rises in left atrial and pulmonary pressures and induce pulmonary edema and right heart failure. Increased left atrial pressure should be maintained as acute decreases can lead to disproportionate drops in ventricular filling. However, overaggressive fluid administration in the setting of already increased left atrial pressure can lead to pulmonary edema. Consequently, tight control of vascular tone and intravascular volume is necessary to avoid dangerous decreases in stroke volume on the one hand and pulmonary edema on the other.

Patients with increased pulmonary artery pressures require special consideration. Changes that can exacerbate pulmonary hypertension, such as hypercarbia, hypoxemia, and hypothermia, need to be avoided and pharmacologic measures to decrease pulmonary vascular resistance should be considered. Similarly, right heart function should be supported as needed with inotropes, and maneuvers that may compromise right heart function (eg, overaggressive fluid administration) should be avoided.

Whenever possible, patients should be medically optimized before proceeding with surgery. Medical management typically involves rate and rhythm control with β-blockers or calcium channel blockers, avoidance of intravascular volume overload with diuretics, and anticoagulation for patients at risk for left atrial thrombus formation.[27] In general, these medications should be continued in the perioperative period. Management of anticoagulation perioperatively should balance risks of bleeding with the risk of thrombosis and systemic embolization and should be discussed in conjunction with the surgeon and internist when feasible. Patients on pulmonary vasodilators should continue these medications because abrupt withdrawal can exacerbate pulmonary hypertension, particularly with inhaled agents.[31,32] Current ACC/AHA guidelines do not recommend endocarditis prophylaxis for patients with isolated mitral stenosis undergoing surgical procedures.[17]

Preoperative administration of anticholinergics is not recommended as the resulting tachycardia is poorly tolerated in this patient population. Preoperative sedation and anxiolysis offer the benefit of controlling stress and concomitant tachycardia, although care must be taken to avoid hypotension, which can dramatically decrease left ventricular preload and respiratory depression, which may exacerbate pulmonary hypertension. For symptomatic patients, continuous hemodynamic monitoring and supplemental oxygen administration are prudent safety measures, especially if the patient is to receive preoperative sedation.

The choice of anesthetic technique should be made on a case-by-case basis. General, neuraxial,[33] and regional techniques may all be used safely, provided that acute drops in preload and tachycardia are avoided. When neuraxial anesthesia is chosen, American Society of Regional Anesthesia and Pain Medicine (ASRA) guidelines for the anticoagulated patient should be adhered to when applicable.[34] Incremental dosing with an epidural catheter offers the potential benefit of controlling the level of sympathectomy and the associated drop in preload. If general anesthesia is selected, induction drugs that have minimal effect on HR and preload (eg, etomidate, narcotics) should be chosen. Thiopental and propofol are probably best avoided because of their direct and indirect effects on ventricular preload. Ketamine is probably best avoided because of its associated tachycardia. Succinylcholine and the nondepolarizing muscle relaxants are acceptable choices, although pancuronium should probably be avoided because of its potential to induce tachycardia. Ensuring an adequate depth of anesthesia before instrumentation of the airway is essential if a tachycardic response is to be avoided. Short-acting β-blockers such as esmolol should be on hand to prevent and treat breakthrough tachycardia. Defibrillator paddles or pads should be available for all patients with mitral stenosis, particularly for those in sinus rhythm, as conversion to atrial fibrillation can lead to rapid hemodynamic deterioration and may necessitate immediate cardioversion. In patients with pulmonary hypertension, it is of utmost importance to avoid even brief periods of hypoxemia and hypercarbia as these can lead to further increases in pulmonary pressures and acute right ventricular failure. Maintenance of anesthesia can be achieved with inhalational or intravenous techniques. Special care must be taken to provide a sufficient depth of anesthesia to blunt the sympathetic response to surgery and the accompanying tachycardia, and to avoid excessive vasodilation and cardiac depression.

Standard monitors recommended by the ASA should always be used. Invasive arterial blood pressure monitoring should be instituted before induction of anesthesia to allow for rapid detection and treatment of decreases in blood pressure. Central venous access allows continuous monitoring of right atrial pressures and a conduit for pressor and inotrope administration. If central venous pressure is being used to titrate intravenous fluid administration, patients with advanced mitral stenosis may have increased right atrial pressures secondary to chronic pulmonary hypertension, tricuspid regurgitation, or both, therefore the central venous pressure trend should be used in this setting in lieu of the absolute number. Although direct clinical benefit has never been shown, PACs are potentially useful, particularly in patients with pulmonary hypertension or right ventricular dysfunction. PACs allow direct measurement of pulmonary artery pressure, pulmonary vascular resistance, left atrial pressure, SVR, CO, and mixed venous oxygen saturation. If left atrial pressures are being measured it is critical to recognize that they will be increased secondary to the stenotic mitral valve and can therefore overestimate true LV preload. Continuous TEE offers the advantage of real-time visualization of right and left ventricular function, filling, and estimation of pulmonary artery pressures. However, it requires a high level of expertise and is labor intensive. Current ACC/AHA guidelines give a class IIa indication for intraoperative TEE monitoring in patients at risk for hemodynamic compromise.[20]

Managing intraoperative changes in hemodynamics and intravascular fluid status in patients with mitral stenosis can be challenging. Abrupt decreases in SVR must be treated immediately as left ventricular filling depends on increased left atrial pressures. Pure α agonists such as phenylephrine effectively raise SVR and have the added benefit of a reflex decrease in HR, although they can exacerbate pulmonary hypertension. Limited data with arginine vasopressin suggest that bolus use of the drug in patients with low SVR and pulmonary hypertension results in increased SVR with minimal effects on pulmonary pressures.[35] Fluid replacement should be carefully titrated as overzealous administration can lead to pulmonary edema, pulmonary hypertension, and acute right heart dysfunction, whereas failure to replace losses can lead to exaggerated drops in left ventricular preload and CO. Right ventricular dysfunction in the setting of pulmonary hypertension should be treated with inotropic support and pulmonary vasodilation. Agents that have inotropic and pulmonary vasodilatory effects (dobutamine, milrinone) may be ideal. When drugs with significant β-adrenergic activity are used, care must be taken to avoid tachycardia. Although data regarding use of inhaled pulmonary vasodilator in patients with mitral stenosis are scant, available evidence suggests that use of these drugs in this population decreases pulmonary vascular resistance without detrimental effects on left ventricular preload.[36]

As on induction, HR and blood pressure should be carefully monitored and controlled on emergence from anesthesia. Reversal of neuromuscular blockade and concomitant use of anticholinergics pose a particular risk. In the future, reversal with novel agents like sugammadex may allow for reversal of neuromuscular blockade without causing tachycardia.[37] Use of topical laryngotracheal or intravenous lidocaine near the end of the procedure may blunt the response to the endotracheal tube on emergence.[38] Ensuring adequate pain control before emergence can also help attenuate emergence phenomena and sympathetic response to pain in the early postoperative period.

Postoperative care should continue to focus on the same hemodynamic goals discussed earlier. Patients with symptomatic disease who undergo open intra-abdominal or intrathoracic procedures should be considered for postoperative admission to the intensive care unit to ensure the most attentive care. Patients who are started on inhaled pulmonary vasodilators (particularly nitric oxide) intraoperatively should not have the drug discontinued abruptly without a formal weaning program because of the risk of rebound pulmonary hypertension.[27] Patients at risk for left atrial thrombus formation and systemic embolization should have their anticoagulant medications restarted as soon as the immediate risk of bleeding has passed.

MITRAL REGURGITATION
Epidemiology

Mitral regurgitation is the most commonly encountered valvular abnormality in the general population. Trace or mild regurgitation is frequently encountered in healthy individuals.[39] Clinically significant (moderate and severe) disease occurs often also, with an overall prevalence of 1.7%. The incidence of moderate and severe disease increases with age, peaking at 9.3% in those more than 75 years of age. It is estimated that in the United States there are 2 to 2.5 million people with moderate to severe mitral regurgitation.[1]

Cause

There are multiple causes of mitral regurgitation, including myxomatous degeneration, ischemic disease, endocarditis, rheumatic disease, trauma, and congenital abnormalities. Myxomatous degeneration accounts for most cases (>60%) that present for surgical repair.[40] Ischemic mitral regurgitation probably accounts for most moderate/severe disease in the general population.[41]

Pathophysiology

Mitral regurgitation can present in acute and chronic forms. In acute mitral regurgitation, sudden development of severe insufficiency (typically from papillary muscle rupture or endocarditis) in the setting of a relatively noncompliant left atrium results in dramatic increases in left atrial, pulmonary venous, and pulmonary arterial pressures. These patients typically present in extremis and require immediate surgical intervention. Patients with severe, acute mitral regurgitation rarely present for noncardiac surgery. The remainder of this section focuses on chronic mitral regurgitation, which is commonly encountered in patients presenting for noncardiac surgery.

The mechanisms of mitral regurgitation can be divided into functional and organic categories. In functional disease mitral regurgitation occurs in the setting of a structurally normal valve (ie, regurgitation secondary to postischemic ventricular remodeling), whereas in organic disease leaflet abnormalities (ie, leaflet prolapse secondary to myxomatous degeneration) cause regurgitation (**Fig. 4**).[42] In cases of functional regurgitation, mitral insufficiency typically occurs in the setting of an already impaired and dilated LV and concomitant enlarged left atrium with increased left atrial pressures.

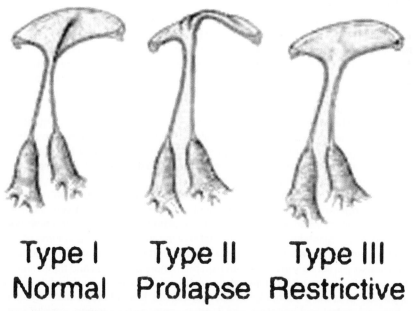

Type I   Type II   Type III
Normal   Prolapse   Restrictive

Fig. 4. Basic abnormalities of the mitral valve seen in patients with mitral regurgitation. Type I: normal leaflet function, as seen in patients with functional MR. Type II: leaflet prolapse, as seen in myxomatous degeneration. Type III leaflet restriction as seen in rheumatic MR. (*From* Lawrie GM. Mitral valve repair versus replacement. Current recommendations and long term results. Cardiol Clin 1998;16:438; with permission.)

The regurgitant volume causes further increases in left atrial and pulmonary pressures. In addition, mitral regurgitation leads to a volume-overloaded LV and consequently increases the risk of heart failure when ventricular function is already compromised. Chronic functional mitral regurgitation may contribute to further left ventricular dysfunction and ventricular and atrial remodeling (dilatation).[43] This situation results in a vicious cycle whereby ventricular impairment and remodeling lead to functional regurgitation and functional regurgitation in turn hastens the progression of ventricular impairment and remodeling.

In organic mitral regurgitation, left ventricular function is typically normal at the onset of disease. As mitral valve function progressively deteriorates, left-sided volume overload ensues, leading to left atrial and left ventricular remodeling. Left ventricular remodeling causes a thin-walled, dilated ventricle, which results initially in improved diastolic function and maximizes stroke volume to assist in unloading the heart.[44] Left atrial remodeling results in an enlarged and compliant chamber, the better to receive regurgitant flow without resulting in dangerous increases in left atrial and right-sided pressures. Left ventricular function is typically well preserved until well into the course of disease and increases in pulmonary pressure are typically modest because of increased left atrial compliance. However, as the disease progresses, these compensatory mechanisms fail and systolic and diastolic ventricular function are impaired. In addition, it is crucial to appreciate that because of the regurgitant lesion, effective impedance to ejection is reduced, even in the setting of a normal measured afterload. Consequently, ventricular dysfunction may be present even in the setting of a normal-appearing ejection fraction.[24]

Anesthetic Considerations

Patients with severe or symptomatic mitral regurgitation should be carefully evaluated and optimized before noncardiac surgery whenever possible.[3] Ideally, candidates for mitral valve reconstruction, replacement, or percutaneous valvuloplasty should have these procedures performed before proceeding with elective surgery. This section focuses on the perioperative management of patients with mitral regurgitation who are not candidates for the procedures outlined earlier or those who are presenting for emergency surgery.

Perioperative hemodynamic goals in patients with significant mitral regurgitation are predicated on maximizing true left ventricular output (volume ejected across the AV) and minimizing regurgitant flow (volume ejected retrograde across the mitral valve). In patients without ischemic heart disease, these goals are best accomplished by a combination of afterload reduction and support of relatively high HRs. Reducing afterload increases effective CO by decreasing impedance to left ventricular flow. As blood is preferentially directed to the systemic circulation during ventricular ejection, the regurgitant volume is decreased. Increasing HR (typically to the high normal range) decreases diastolic time, thereby decreasing the interval and volume of regurgitation. These maneuvers become even more important in patients with decompensated disease, particularly in those with high pulmonary pressures and right ventricular dysfunction. Patients with significant coronary artery disease and ischemic mitral regurgitation present a particular challenge, as the low afterload and higher HRs that improve mitral regurgitation can lead to myocardial oxygen supply/demand mismatch by increasing myocardial demand (increased HR) and decreasing coronary blood flow (decreasing afterload and diastolic coronary perfusion time). In addition, aggravating coronary ischemia may also worsen the mitral regurgitation by compromising papillary muscle function. In these cases, maintaining normal afterload and a low normal HR may be advisable, despite the effects that these maneuvers may have on regurgitant volume.

Whenever possible, patients should be medically optimized before proceeding with surgery. Medical management of mitral regurgitation is complicated by the high incidence of concomitant atrial fibrillation. In some series, more than 50% of patients presenting for surgical intervention have chronic atrial fibrillation.[45] These patients are often receiving agents to help control ventricular rate (β-blockers, calcium channel blockers), which should be continued through the perioperative period. Patients in atrial fibrillation are typically placed on anticoagulants because of the increased risk of embolic stroke. Management of anticoagulation perioperatively should balance the risk of bleeding with the risk of thrombosis and systemic embolization. These concerns should be discussed in conjunction with the surgeon and internist, when feasible. Patients with mitral regurgitation may be receiving afterload-reducing drugs. Some of these drugs (angiotensin-converting enzyme [ACE] inhibitors, angiotensin receptor blockers [ARBs]) have been associated with hypotension under general anesthesia.[46] However, no recommendations for cessation before anesthesia have been adopted. Current ACC/AHA guidelines do not recommend endocarditis prophylaxis for patients with isolated mitral regurgitation undergoing surgical procedures unless there is a prior history of endocarditis, congenital heart disease, or a structurally abnormal valve following heart transplantation.[13]

Preoperative sedation and anticholinergics are usually well tolerated in patients with mitral regurgitation. In patients with regurgitation secondary to active coronary artery disease anticholinergics are probably best avoided as the resultant tachycardia can induce myocardial ischemia. In patients with pulmonary hypertension, sedation should be used cautiously because hypercarbia and hypoxia secondary to respiratory depression can lead to further increases in pulmonary arterial pressure.

General and regional anesthetic techniques, including neuraxial anesthesia, are considered safe in patients with mitral regurgitation. If neuraxial blockade is to be used ASRA guidelines for the anticoagulated patient should be adhered to when applicable.[15] The sympathectomy and resultant afterload reduction observed after neuraxial block can help decrease regurgitant volume, as described earlier. Similarly, most intravenous and inhalational anesthetics can be used safely, as afterload reduction in this patient population is beneficial. Patients with ischemic mitral regurgitation with myocardium at risk may not tolerate afterload reduction and increased HRs. Anesthetic agents that preserve afterload without increasing HR (etomidate, narcotics) may be better choices for these patients. Patients with pulmonary hypertension and right heart dysfunction may be preload dependent. Agents that acutely drop preload (thiopental) are best avoided in this subgroup of patients.

Standard monitors recommended by the ASA should always be used and are adequate for most patients with mild disease. Invasive arterial blood pressure monitoring should be considered in patients with moderate or severe disease and for those with underlying coronary artery disease, pulmonary hypertension, or ventricular dysfunction. Central venous access allows continuous monitoring of right atrial pressures and a conduit for pressor and inotrope administration and should be considered in these patients also. If central venous pressure is being used to titrate intravenous fluid administration, patients with advanced mitral regurgitation may have increased right atrial pressures secondary to chronic pulmonary hypertension, tricuspid regurgitation, or both. As a consequence, the central venous pressure trend should be used to direct fluid replacement in lieu of the absolute number. Although direct clinical benefit has never been shown, PACs are potentially useful, particularly in patients with pulmonary hypertension or right ventricular dysfunction. PACs allow direct measurement of pulmonary artery pressure, pulmonary vascular resistance, left atrial pressure, SVR, CO, and mixed venous oxygen saturation. In patients with isolated mitral regurgitation, right-sided CO measured by thermodilution overestimates effective left ventricular output. Measures of left-sided output (eg, esophageal Doppler monitoring, arterial pressure waveform analysis) may provide a more accurate reflection of left heart output, although data regarding these monitors in patients with mitral regurgitation are currently lacking.[47,48] Continuous TEE offers the advantage of real-time visualization of right and left ventricular function, filling, and estimation of pulmonary artery pressures. However, it requires a high level of expertise and is labor intensive. Current ACC/AHA guidelines give a class IIa indication for intraoperative TEE monitoring in patients at risk for hemodynamic compromise.[16]

Intraoperative changes in hemodynamics and intravascular fluid status in patients with mitral regurgitation can be managed effectively, if the general hemodynamic goals for these patients are respected. Abrupt decreases in SVR can be treated with mixed α and β agonists like ephedrine, as pure α agonists increase afterload and cause a reflex drop in HR, thereby theoretically increasing regurgitation. Fluid replacement should be carefully titrated, as overzealous administration can lead to pulmonary edema, pulmonary hypertension, and acute right heart dysfunction. In patients with ischemic mitral regurgitation a decrease in afterload that results in a deterioration of hemodynamics (ie, increased left atrial or pulmonary arterial pressures) may imply myocardial ischemia or worsening ischemic regurgitation. Such derangements should be treated initially with measures to increase coronary perfusion (decrease HR and increase afterload). If these maneuvers fail, and the patient continues to deteriorate, consideration should be given to placement of an intra-aortic balloon pump (IABP),[49] as counterpulsation increases coronary perfusion and decreases left ventricular afterload. Right ventricular dysfunction in the setting of pulmonary hypertension should be treated with inotropic support, pulmonary vasodilation, and measures to decrease the regurgitant fraction. Agents that have inotropic and vasodilatory effects (milrinone) may be ideal. Consideration of placement of an IABP is warranted if other, more conventional measures seem to be unsuccessful.[50] Although reports of the successful use of inhaled pulmonary vasodilators in patients with pulmonary hypertension following mitral valve surgery abound,[51] evidence supporting their use in patients with severe regurgitation undergoing noncardiac surgery is lacking.

During emergence from anesthesia, efforts should be made to avoid periods of hypertension that can worsen regurgitation. In patients with ischemic mitral regurgitation tachycardia should be avoided when possible and treated with short-acting β-blockers as needed. In patients with pulmonary hypertension, it is important to recognize and manage respiratory insufficiency on emergence as hypoxia and hypercarbia can lead to further increases in pulmonary pressure and right ventricular decompensation.

Evidence suggests that the early postoperative period poses an especially high risk to patients with moderate/severe mitral regurgitation.[52] During the early postoperative course following major surgery, patients with significant disease need to be observed for signs of pulmonary edema, respiratory insufficiency, and arrhythmias, which occur frequently. In patients with complicated disease (coronary artery disease, pulmonary hypertension) or anticipated ongoing fluid shifts, transfer to an intensive care unit for further monitoring in the immediate postoperative period should be considered.

SUMMARY

Left-sided valvular heart lesions present a myriad of potential difficulties during perioperative care for noncardiac surgery. A thorough understanding of the pathophysiology of the presenting lesion along with its implications in the perioperative period is crucial in preventing undesirable outcomes. Patients with left-sided valvular disease require careful preoperative evaluation, optimization and planning, vigilant intraoperative monitoring, and tight hemodynamic control that must be continued into the postoperative period when appropriate. As the population continues to age, we can expect to treat rising numbers of patients with these derangements, making it more crucial than ever to be prepared for these encounters.

REFERENCES

1. Nkomo VT, Gardin JM, Skelton TM, et al. Burden of valvular heart diseases: a population based study. Lancet 2006;368:1005–11.
2. Goldman L, Caldera DL, Nussbaum SR, et al. Multifactorial index of cardiac risk in noncardiac surgical procedures. N Engl J Med 1977;297(16):845–50.
3. Fleisher LA, Beckman JA, Brown KA, et al. ACC/AHA 2007 guidelines on perioperative cardiovascular evaluation and care for noncardiac surgery. J Am Coll Cardiol 2007;50:e159–242.
4. Stewart BF, Siscovick D, Lind BK, et al. Clinical factors associated with calcific aortic valve disease. J Am Coll Cardiol 1997;29:630–4.
5. Pellika PA, Sarano ME, Nishimura RA, et al. Outcome of 622 adults with asymptomatic, hemodynamically significant aortic stenosis during prolonged follow-up. Circulation 2005;111:3290–5.
6. Detsky AS, Anrams HB, Forbath N, et al. Cardiac assessment for patients undergoing noncardiac surgery. A multifactorial clinical risk index. Arch Intern Med 1986;146:2131–4.
7. O'Keefe JH, Shub C, Rettke SR. Risk of noncardiac surgical procedures in patients with aortic stenosis. Mayo Clin Proc 1989;64:400–5.
8. Yarmush L. Noncardiac surgery in the patient with valvular heart disease. Anesthesiol Clin North America 1997;15:69–89.
9. Selzer A. Changing aspects of the natural history of valvular aortic stenosis. N Engl J Med 1987;317:91–8.
10. Roberts WC, Ko JM. Frequency of decades of unicuspid, bicuspid and tricuspid aortic valves in adults having isolated aortic valve replacement for aortic stenosis, with or without associated aortic regurgitation. Circulation 2005;111:920–5.
11. Lindroos M, Kupari M, Heikkila J, et al. Prevalence of aortic valve abnormalities in the elderly: an echocardiographic study of a random population. J Am Coll Cardiol 1993;21:1220–5.
12. Carabello BA. Aortic stenosis. N Engl J Med 2002;346:677–82.
13. Otto CM. Valvular aortic stenosis: disease severity and timing of intervention. J Am Coll Cardiol 2006;47:2141–51.
14. Barash PG. Clinical anesthesia. 5th edition. Philadelphia (PA): Lippincott Williams Wilkins; 2006. 898–901.
15. Mittnacht AJ, Fanshawe M, Konstadt S. Anesthetic considerations in the patient with valvular heart disease undergoing noncardiac surgery. Semin Cardiothorac Vasc Anesth 2008;12:33–59.
16. Hess OM, Villari B, Krayenbuehl HB. Diastolic dysfunction in aortic stenosis. Circulation 1993;87(Suppl 5):73–6.
17. Torsher L, Shub C, Rettke SR, et al. Risk of patients with severe aortic stenosis undergoing noncardiac surgery. Am J Cardiol 1998;81:448–52.

18. Nishimura RA, Carabello BA, Faxon DP, et al. ACC/AHA 2008 guideline update on valvular heart disease: focused update on infective endocarditis. J Am Coll Cardiol 2008;52:676–85.

19. Colard CD, Eappen S, Lynch EP, et al. Continuous spinal anesthesia with invasive hemodynamic monitoring for surgical repair of the hip in two patients with severe aortic stenosis. Anesth Analg 1995;81:195–8.

20. Van Helder T, Smedstad KG. Combined spinal epidural anesthesia in a primigravida with valvular heart disease. Can J Anaesth 1998;45:488–90.

21. Cheitlin MD, Armstrong WF, Aurigemma GP, et al. ACC/AHA/ASE 2003 guideline update for the clinical application of echocardiography: summary article. J Am Soc Echocardiogr 2003;16:1091–110.

22. Berkeredjian R, Grayburn PA. Valvular heart disease: aortic regurgitation. Circulation 2005;112:125–34.

23. Carabello BA, Crawford FA. Valvular heart disease. N Engl J Med 1997;337: 32–41.

24. Stoelting R. Anesthesia and co-existing disease. 4th edition. Philadelphia (PA): Churchill Livingstone Elsevier; 2002. p. 38–42.

25. Padmavati S. Rheumatic fever and rheumatic heart disease in India at the turn of the century. Indian Heart J 2001;53:35–7.

26. Golbasi Z, Ucar O, Keles T, et al. Increased levels of high sensitivity C-reactive protein in patients with chronic rheumatic valve disease: evidence of ongoing inflammation. Eur J Heart Fail 2002;4:593–5.

27. Chandrashekhar Y, Westaby S, Narula J. Mitral stenosis. Lancet 2009;374: 1271–83.

28. Vincelj J, Sokol I, Jaksic O. Prevalence and clinical significance of left atrial spontaneous echo contrast detected by transesophageal echocardiography. Echocardiography 2002;19:319–24.

29. Gash AK, Carabello BA, Cepin D, et al. Left ventricular ejection performance and systolic muscle function in patients with mitral stenosis. Circulation 1983;67:148–54.

30. Diker E, Aydogdu S, Ozdemir M, et al. Prevalence and predictors of atrial fibrillation in rheumatic valvular heart disease. Am J Cardiol 1997;77:96–8.

31. Augoustides JG, Culp K, Smith S. Rebound pulmonary hypertension and cardiogenic shock after withdrawal of inhaled prostacyclin. Anesthesiology 2004;100: 1023–5.

32. Miller OI, Tang SF, Keech A, et al. Rebound pulmonary hypertension on withdrawal of inhaled nitric oxide. Lancet 1995;346:51–2.

33. Pan PH, D'Angelo R. Anesthetic and analgesic management of mitral stenosis during pregnancy. Reg Anesth Pain Med 2004;29:610–5.

34. Holocker TT, Wedel DJ, Benzon H, et al. Regional anesthesia in the anticoagulated patient: defining the risks (the second ASRA Consensus Conference on Neuraxial Anesthesia and Anticoagulation). Reg Anesth Pain Med 2003;28:172–97.

35. Tayama E, Ueda T, Shojima T, et al. Arginine vasopressin is an ideal drug after cardiac surgery for the management of low systemic vascular resistant hypotension concomitant with pulmonary hypertension. Interact Cardiovasc Thorac Surg 2007;6:715–9.

36. Mahoney PD, Loh E, Blitz LR, et al. Hemodynamic effects of inhaled nitric oxide in women with mitral stenosis and pulmonary hypertension. Am J Cardiol 2001;87: 188–92.

37. Sacan O, White PF, Tufanogullari B, et al. Sugammadex reversal of rocuronium induced neuromuscular blockade: a comparison with neostigmine-glycopyrrolate and edophonium-atropine. Anesth Analg 2007;104:569–74.

38. Fagan C, Frizelle HP, Laffey J, et al. The effects of intracuff lidocaine on endotracheal tube induced emergence phenomena after general anesthesia. Anesth Analg 2000;91:201–5.
39. Klein A, Burstow D, Tajik A, et al. Age-related prevalence of valvular regurgitation in normal subjects: a comprehensive color flow examination of 118 volunteers. J Am Soc Echocardiogr 1990;3:54–63.
40. Olson L, Subramanian R, Ackerman D, et al. Surgical pathology of the mitral valve: a study of 712 cases spanning 21 years. Mayo Clin Proc 1987;62:22–34.
41. Marwick TH, Lancelloti P, Pierard L. Ischemic mitral regurgitation: mechanisms and diagnosis. Heart 2009;95:1711–8.
42. Lawrie GM. Mitral valve repair vs replacement. Current recommendations and long-term results. Cardiol Clin 1998;16:437–48.
43. Enriquez-Sarano M, Akins CW, Vahanian A. Mitral regurgitation. Lancet 2009;373:1382–94.
44. Carabello BA. The current therapy for mitral regurgitation. J Am Coll Cardiol 2009;52:319–26.
45. Gillinov AM. Ablation of atrial fibrillation with mitral valve surgery. Curr Opin Cardiol 2005;20:107–14.
46. Comfere T, Sprung J, Kumar MM, et al. Angiotensin system inhibitors in a general surgical population. Anesth Analg 2005;100:636–44.
47. Mayer J, Boldt J, Poland R, et al. Continuous arterial pressure waveform based cardiac output using the FloTrac/Vigileo: a review and meta analysis. J Cardiothorac Vasc Anesth 2009;23:401–6.
48. Schober P, Loer SA, Schwarte LA. Perioperative hemodynamic monitoring with transesophageal Doppler technology. Anesth Analg 2009;109:340–53.
49. Siu SC, Kowalchuk GJ, Welty FK, et al. Intra-aortic balloon counterpulsation supporting the high-risk cardiac patient undergoing urgent non-cardiac surgery. Chest 1991;99:1342–5.
50. Jett GK, Picone AL, Clark RE. Circulatory support for right ventricular dysfunction. J Thorac Cardiovasc Surg 1987;94:95–103.
51. Healy DG, Veerasingam D, McHale J, et al. Successful perioperative utilization of inhaled nitric oxide in mitral valve surgery. J Cardiovasc Surg 2006;47:217–20.
52. Lai HC, Lee WL, Wang KY, et al. Mitral regurgitation complicates postoperative outcome of noncardiac surgery. Am Heart J 2007;153:712–7.

The Intraoperative Management of Patients with Pericardial Tamponade

Christopher J. O'Connor, MD*, Kenneth J. Tuman, MD

KEYWORDS

• Pericardial tamponade • Pericardial effusion
• Pericardial window • Shock

The anesthetic management of patients with pericardial tamponade is challenging, as they present with not only the cardiovascular compromise that defines pericardial tamponade, but often have comorbid conditions that increase the complexity of their management. This review describes the pathophysiology, etiology, clinical presentation, and anesthetic management of patients with pericardial tamponade, with an emphasis on the intraoperative period and the management of pericardial window procedures, the most common clinical scenario where anesthesiologists will encounter pericardial tamponade.

ANATOMY AND PHYSIOLOGY OF THE NORMAL PERICARDIUM

The pericardial sac consists of 2 layers—visceral and parietal—that envelop the heart. The visceral pericardium is tightly adherent to the heart and reflects back toward the base of the great vessels while forming the inner layer of the parietal pericardium.[1] These pericardial reflections around the great vessels produce 2 potential spaces that are frequently evident by transesophageal echocardiography (TEE): the oblique and transverse sinuses. The pericardial sac normally contains up to 50 mL of serous fluid that minimizes friction on the epicardium and equalizes hydrostatic pressures over the surface of the heart.[2] Although the pericardium is not essential for normal cardiac function, it serves several useful physiologic purposes: it limits

---

The authors have received no external funding for this project.
Department of Anesthesiology, Rush University Medical Center, 1653 West Congress Parkway, Chicago, IL 60612, USA
* Corresponding author.
E-mail address: cjoconnormd@sbcglobal.net

Anesthesiology Clin 28 (2010) 87–96
doi:10.1016/j.anclin.2010.01.011   anesthesiology.theclinics.com
1932-2275/10/$ – see front matter. Published by Elsevier Inc.

distention of the cardiac chambers and facilitates ventriculoatrial coupling[1]; its liga-mentous attachments maintain the heart in a relatively fixed position in the chest; and it contributes to regulation of coronary tone via prostaglandin release and neural innervations.[2]

This restraining effect of the pericardium is best demonstrated in its structural prop-erties, which have been likened to that of rubber, in that at low cardiac filling pressures, the tissue is elastic and expands.[2] However, due to a relatively nonlinear pressure-volume relationship (**Fig. 1**) and noncompliant tissue, as volume in the pericardial sac increases, the pressure increases abruptly (see **Fig. 1**) and exerts this pressure on the surface of the heart, which is, in turn, transmitted to the intracardiac chambers, resulting in increased cardiac filling pressures (ie, the central venous and pulmonary artery occlusion pressures [CVP and PAOP, respectively]). Thus, the pericardium has a small reserve volume and once that critical volume is reached, intrapericardial and intracardiac filling pressures increase and the diastolic volumes decrease dramat-ically, impairing cardiac filling and reducing cardiac output. In contrast, chronic stretching of the pericardial sac due to gradual accumulation of fluid results in a more compliant pericardium and therefore slowly accumulating but large pericardial effusions may not produce tamponade, while acutely increased fluid collections are more likely to produce tamponade with much smaller fluid volumes (see **Fig. 1**).[1] This altered compliance is likely due to growth of pericardial tissue in response to chronic stretching.[2] These changes are more dramatic for the thin-walled right atrium and ventricle (RA and RV, respectively), which have lower pressures and less muscular tissue than the left ventricle (LV).

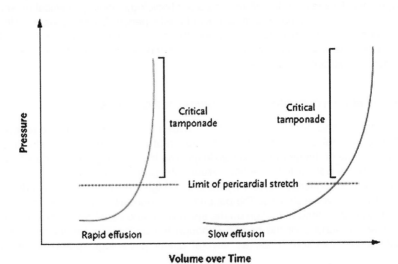

Fig. 1. The pressure-volume relationship of the pericardial sac in both acute and chronic pericardial effusions. In rapidly accumulating fluid collections in the pericardial sac, as in acute tamponade, once the critical reserve volume of the pericardium is exceeded the pericardial pressure rises rapidly, quickly exceeding those of the right heart chambers and leading to right heart chamber collapse. In contrast, with chronically accumulating effusions, large volumes may only produce modest increases in pericardial pressure. This alteration of the compliance of the pericardial sac has been attributed to "stretching" of the visceral and parietal layers of the pericardium. (*Reprinted from* Spodick DH. Acute cardiac tamponade. N Engl J Med 2003;349:684–90; with permission. Copyright © 2003, Massachusetts Medical Society.)

ETIOLOGY

The etiology of pericardial effusions is extensive. Virtually any infectious or inflammatory condition can produce a significant pericardial effusion, and clotted and nonclotted blood, pus, serous fluid, or chyle can produce pericardial tamponade. **Box 1** demonstrates the different causes of pericardial effusions and pericardial tamponade. The disease states representing patients who present for surgical pericardial window procedures are less extensive.

PERICARDIAL TAMPONADE
Etiology

As noted in **Box 1**, there are numerous causes of pericardial effusions, but few progress to overt tamponade. Those disease states with a high frequency of progression to tamponade include bacterial and fungal infections, and malignancies. In an analysis of 105 cases of patients undergoing pericardial window surgery at the authors' institution, the most common causes of large pericardial effusions requiring pericardial window surgery included effusions associated with malignancy or end-stage renal disease (ESRD), effusions observed 3 to 7 days after cardiac surgery, and idiopathic effusions (CJ O'Connor, MD, unpublished data, 2010). Direct chest trauma, ruptured ascending aortic aneurysms, and effusions secondary to percutaneous cardiac interventions[3] are all conditions whereby tamponade is acute, life-threatening, and requires immediate surgical intervention and repair. Pericardial effusions are common after cardiac surgery, although acute tamponade is most often observed immediately after surgery in the intensive care unit; delayed tamponade is less frequent, but still a concern.[4–7] Pepi and colleagues[6] observed pericardial effusions in 64% of 780 consecutive patients undergoing cardiac surgery and were more common after

---

Box 1
Etiology of pericardial tamponade

Common

- Idiopathic
- Iatrogenic (postcardiac surgery/invasive cardiac procedure, including percutaneous coronary intervention, electrophysiologic procedure, percutaneous valve repair)
- Trauma
- Malignancy
- End-stage renal disease

Uncommon

- Collagen vascular disease (ie, lupus, scleroderma, and so forth)
- Tuberculosis
- Postmyocardial infarction
- Bacterial infection
- Aortic dissection
- Radiation

Data from Meltser H, Kalaria V. Cardiac tamponade. Catheter Cardiovasc Interv 2005;64:245–55.

coronary artery surgery than following valve procedures. The effusions were loculated in 58% and diffuse in the remaining. Ninety-eight percent were classified as mild to moderate in size and did not require intervention. In contrast, approximately 2% were large, most were receiving anticoagulants, and all developed tamponade, ultimately requiring drainage procedures.[6] Tamponade developed early (<10 days postoperatively) in 6 patients and late (postoperative days 14–23) in the remaining 9 patients, and was more often encountered after valve surgery. Effusions are also seen after cardiac transplantation,[7] and although the majority resolve, almost 10% in one clinical series developed tamponade that required drainage. Size discrepancy between the donor heart and a larger recipient mediastinum may also favor exudation of fluid into the pericardial space.[7] Acute postoperative pericardial tamponade may also be more common in procedures associated with significant intraoperative hemorrhage, such as ascending aortic aneurysm resection or left ventricular assist device procedures, although this has yet to be quantitatively analyzed.

ESRD is often associated with pericarditis and pericardial effusions.[8,9] This phenomenon has been termed either uremic pericarditis, seen in patients before or soon after the initiation of dialytic therapy, or dialysis pericarditis, applied to patients who develop pericardial involvement more than 8 weeks after initiation of dialysis.[8] The incidence of dialysis pericarditis ranges from 2% to 21% and pericardial tamponade occurs in 14% to 56% of this group of patients,[8,9] whereas patients with uremic pericarditis and pericardial effusions appear to respond to aggressive hemodialysis and to require drainage less frequently. Patients with moderate to large effusions associated with pericardial tamponade always required pericardial window surgery. Dialysis-related effusions were one of the more common causes of pericardial window surgery in the authors' own analysis, although the chronic nature of the disease and the frequent presence of coexisting hypertension rarely appears to lead to significant hypotension, so that general anesthesia is typically well tolerated in this group of patients.

Pathophysiology

Given the small reserve volume of the pericardial sac, relatively small but rapid accumulation of fluid can have dramatic effects on cardiac preload, cardiac output, and blood pressure. In contrast, large, chronic effusions that have progressed slowly are frequently well tolerated and typically do not show evidence of chamber collapse due to the stretching effect of the pericardial sac (see **Fig. 1**).[10] In either case, when the pericardial pressure reaches a critical stage, the effusion reduces the volume of the cardiac chambers, increases intracavitary pressures, drastically reduces cardiac preload, and reduces cardiac output.[2] Despite large increases in intracardiac pressures, the transmural pressures and intracardiac volumes are decreased. In contrast to the normal biphasic nature of venous return, venous return becomes confined to systole in severe tamponade and ceases during diastole, when intrapericardial pressures are maximal and equal to right and left atrial (LA) and left ventricular end-diastolic pressures (typically 15–20 mm Hg). Systolic function remains normal or even hyperdynamic, although bulging of the interventricular septum into the LV and systemic hypotension may impair systolic function and coronary perfusion.[1,10,11] Elevated pericardial pressure primarily affects right heart filling, and experimental studies demonstrate right heart compression, as is clearly evident by echocardiography in patients with tamponade.

Clinical findings include tachycardia, dyspnea, diminished arterial and cardiac pulsations and muffled heart tones, complaints of chest discomfort, elevated jugular venous pressures, diaphoresis, pulsus paradoxus (an exaggeration of the normal decrease in blood pressure during inspiration), and hypotension. Compensatory sympathetic nervous system responses produce tachycardia and peripheral vasoconstriction, but when these mechanisms are exhausted, hypotension and a shock state ensue.[1] In chronic effusions, this sympathetic response may occasionally produce systemic hypertension, a hemodynamic picture the authors have frequently observed.

Diagnosis

The electrocardiogram (ECG) typically reveals diffuse low voltage and electrical alternans (**Fig. 2**; affecting all ECG waves or just the QRS complex),[10] although diffuse upsloping ST segment elevation may be seen with acute pericarditis.[12,13] Electrical alternans represents alternating voltage with each cardiac cycle due to anterior-posterior swinging of the heart in the nonconstrained, fluid-filled pericardial sac.[10,14] This phenomenon is observed with alternating heartbeats, such that the heart is physically closer to the chest wall with every other beat, resulting in taller r-waves.[2,14] The chest radiograph shows a normal heart size until the effusion is moderate in size (at least

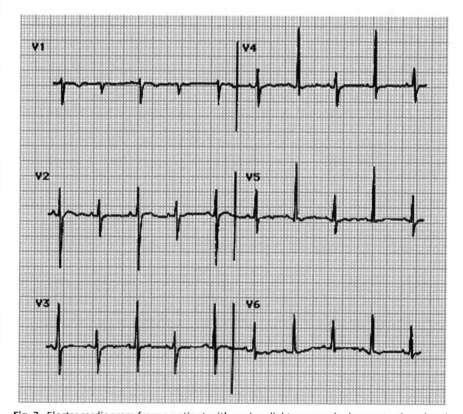

Fig. 2. Electrocardiogram from a patient with pericardial tamponade demonstrating electrical alternans, a phenomenon caused by alternating voltage with each cardiac cycle due to anterior-posterior swinging of the heart in the nonconstrained, fluid-filled pericardial sac. This process is observed with alternating heartbeats, such that the heart is physically closer to the chest wall with every other beat, resulting in taller r-waves. (*Reproduced with permission from* Goldberger AL. Electrocardiogram in pericarditis and pericardial tamponade. In: UpToDate, Basow, DS(Ed), UpToDate, Waltham, MA 2009. Copyright © 2009 UpToData, Inc. For more information visit www.uptodate.com)

>200 mL); thereafter, the cardiac silhouette is enlarged in a flask or water-bottle appearance.[2] Cardiac catheterization, though infrequently performed for diagnostic purposes, demonstrates an attenuated or blunted Y-descent on the RA waveform (normally, the descent in the waveform after the V wave represents opening of the tricuspid valve and early RV diastolic filling) due to diastolic equalization of pressures in the RA and RV and the lack of effective flow in early ventricular diastole[11]; elevation and equalization of filling pressures in all cardiac chambers; varying peak aortic pressures by more than 10 to 12 mm Hg; and decreased cardiac output. Typically, however, echocardiography is the sole cardiovascular diagnostic test performed, although pulmonary artery catheterization (such as in the immediate postoperative period following cardiac surgery) may reveal equilibration of central venous, pulmonary artery, and pulmonary artery occlusion pressures.

Echocardiography is the diagnostic test of choice in establishing the presence of pericardial tamponade. Echocardiographic findings are summarized in **Table 1**. A commonly employed grading system for the size of pericardial effusions defines a small effusion as less than 9 mm; a moderate effusion as 10 to 19 mm; and a large effusion as greater than 20 mm.[6,11] The most characteristic, though not highly specific, echocardiographic signs are chamber collapse, most often the RA and RV, as noted earlier (**Figs. 3** and **4**/Video 1). During early diastole, the RV free wall invaginates and at end-diastole, the RA wall invaginates. RA collapse is very common and is a more sensitive finding when it lasts for at least 30% of the cardiac cycle.[10,15,16] Left atrial collapse occurs in approximately 25% of patients and is very specific for tamponade. As previously noted, echocardiographic findings may be atypical following cardiac surgery, with localized, nonfree-flowing effusions or clot present, along with left atrial collapse. LV collapse is rare due to the muscular nature of the ventricular wall, although bulging of the interventricular septum from the right to the left ventricle is very specific for tamponade (and accounts, in part, for the phenomenon of pulsus paradoxus).[1]

Table 1 Echocardiographic features of pericardial tamponade	
Finding	**Comment**
RA collapse and invagination	100% sensitive for tamponade, but less specific
Left atrial collapse	Very specific for tamponade
RV free wall diastolic collapse	More specific for tamponade
Paradoxic motion of the interventricular septum	More specific for tamponade
Distension of the inferior vena cava	Sensitive but nonspecific; reflects elevated RA pressures
Exaggerated respiratory variations in mitral and tricuspid inflow velocities	Marked inspiratory increase in tricuspid, and decrease in mitral, inflow velocities with inspiration
Large effusion, rotational swinging of the heart	Effusions >20 mm
LV collapse	Rare
Clot or loculated effusions	More common after cardiac surgery

Abbreviations: LV, left ventricular; RA, right atrial; RV, right ventricular.

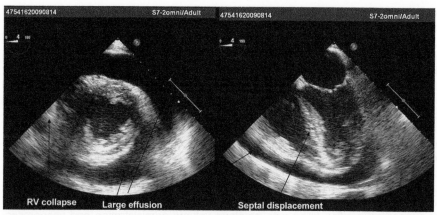

Fig. 3. Intraoperative transesophageal echocardiogram demonstrating a large pericardial effusion in a patient with end-stage renal disease and pericardial tamponade. On the left, a 4-chamber view shows the small right ventricle and the rightward shift of the interventricular septum, a finding very specific for pericardial tamponade. On the right, a transgastric view reveals the large effusion, the small LV, and collapse of the right ventricle, as evidenced by the absence of the right ventricle in the image.

Treatment

The treatment of acute pericardial tamponade typically requires immediate drainage, usually by needle pericardiocentesis using either echocardiographic or fluoroscopic guidance. A catheter can be placed in the pericardial space for several days for continued drainage, and may also allow the instillation of sclerosing agents, corticosteroids, or thrombolytic drugs.[1] Removal of as little as 50 mL of pericardial fluid can commonly produce significant hemodynamic improvement due to the steep pericardial pressure-volume relationship (see **Fig. 1**). Surgical drainage is indicated

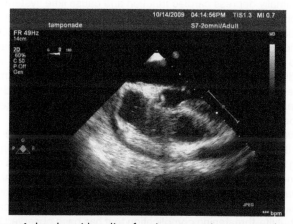

Fig. 4. shot from a 4-chamber video clip of an intraoperative transesophageal echocardiogram from a patient with a large pericardial effusion and pericardial tamponade. Typical inversion and collapse of the right atrium seen with pericardial tamponade is shown. While very sensitive for tamponade, it is less specific than diastolic collapse of the right ventricle. (To see full video go to http://www.anesthesiology.theclinics.com.)

for patients with hemopericardium from acute aortic dissection, penetrating trauma, percutaneous cardiac interventions with ongoing hemorrhage, and ventricular rupture. Large chronic effusions with moderate degrees of tamponade are typically well tolerated and can often be drained on an elective basis. Surgical drainage can be accomplished either via subxiphoid pericardial window creation,[17] a small anterior thoracotomy[18,19] (open or thoracoscopic), or formation of a pericardial-peritoneal window.[20] Surgical drainage allows for digital exploration (useful for evacuating clotted pericardial fluid), pericardial biopsies for diagnostic purposes, and more effective removal of fibrinous debris, especially in the postcardiac surgery setting.[17] Mortality is low and survival is largely dependent on the underlying disease process, which in the majority of published cases is secondary to malignancy, the most common cause associated with large pericardial effusions. Advantages of the subxiphoid approach include its efficacy, simplicity, and ability to be accomplished with local anesthesia, if necessary. Medical therapy for acute tamponade is primarily aimed at supporting cardiac filling with cautious volume administration and vasopressor support until definitive drainage can be accomplished.

Anesthetic Management

The literature contains little evidence-based information regarding the proper anesthetic management of patients with pericardial tamponade. In the absence of tamponade associated with acute aortic dissection or penetrating chest trauma, which requires immediate surgical intervention, the most commonly encountered scenario is the patient presenting for pericardial window formation, either acutely or on an elective basis. For patients who are hemodynamically unstable, pericardial drainage may be accomplished with local anesthetic infiltration and judicious administration of sedative and analgesic agents, such as ketamine,[21] midazolam, or fentanyl. Numerous surgical reports have documented the success of local infiltration in the creation of subxiphoid pericardial windows.[22–24] Alternatively, initial drainage can be accomplished with local anesthetic infiltration, and after hemodynamic improvement, general anesthesia may be induced. If general anesthesia is employed, which may be requested when TEE will be used or following cardiac surgery, common sense dictates selection of induction agents that minimally depress cardiac function and cause little systemic vasodilation and hypotension, such as ketamine and etomidate. Data from 105 patients undergoing pericardial window formation at the authors' institution (CJ O'Connor, MD, unpublished data, 2010) indicate that outcome is no different between patients managed with local anesthesia and sedation and patients receiving general anesthesia, although brief vasopressor administration may be required in the latter group following induction of general anesthesia. Advantages of general anesthesia include improved surgical evacuation of pericardial contents, facilitation of TEE examination for success of surgical evacuation of pericardial contents, and enhanced patient comfort.

Mechanical ventilation may increase pulmonary vascular resistance and decrease RV outflow, further exacerbating leftward septal shift, impairing LV filling, and potentially worsening systemic hypotension. Because of this, some clinicians suggest maintaining spontaneous ventilation. However, merely avoiding large tidal volumes and high peak airway pressures will likely minimize the impact of ventilation on systemic hemodynamics, and allow for general anesthesia and adequate surgical conditions.

An unusual, but life-threatening complication that has been observed following pericardial drainage for tamponade has been pulmonary edema.[25–32] Pulmonary edema appears to occur more frequently after large volume pericardiocentesis and in patients with chronic pericardial effusions. The etiology of pulmonary edema and global LV dysfunction after drainage is unclear, but may be related to a sudden abrupt increase in preload and ventricular filling, increased systolic wall stress,[25] and fluid extravasation into the alveoli and pulmonary interstitium. Myocardial stunning has also been invoked as a possible cause for pulmonary edema, as has volume mismatch in the setting of enhanced sympathetic tone.[25,28] Because of this complication, some clinicians recommend slow decompression of the pericardium over 24 hours with catheter drainage,[26] although this is not pragmatic during pericardial window surgery and, given that removal of very small volumes results in prompt hemodynamic improvement, it also seems impractical and potentially unachievable in these cases. A more significant concern is predrainage volume loading to maintain preload during the time of pericardial tamponade, as is often suggested in textbooks. This action may increase the potential for volume overload after the pericardial fluid is drained, and thus hemodynamic support with temporary vasopressor administration may be more appropriate until definitive drainage can be achieved.

SUMMARY

In conclusion, patients with acute pericardial tamponade will have impaired cardiovascular hemodynamics, and immediate drainage of the pericardial fluid is essential for survival. In contrast, patients with large, chronic effusions due to ESRD or malignancy are often best managed with surgical pericardial window formation under general anesthesia.

APPENDIX: SUPPLEMENTARY MATERIAL

Supplementary material can be found, in the online version, at doi:10.1016/j.anclin. 2010.01.011.

REFERENCES

1. Hoit BD. Pericardial disease and pericardial tamponade. Crit Care Med 2007; 35(Suppl 8):S355–64.
2. LeWinter MM. Pericardial diseases. In: Libby P, Bonow RO, Mann DL, et al, editors. Braunwald's heart disease: a textbook of cardiovascular medicine. 8th edition. Philadelphia: Saunders Elsevier; 2007. p. 1829–54, chapter 70.
3. Chen SW, Liu SW, Lin JX. [Incidence, risk factors and management of pericardial effusion post radiofrequency catheter ablation in patients with atrial fibrillations]. Zhonghua Xin Xue Guan Bing Za Zhi 2008;36(9):801–6 [in Chinese].
4. Bommer WJ, Follette DF, Pollock M, et al. Tamponade in patients undergoing cardiac surgery: a clinical-echocardiographic diagnosis. Am Heart J 1995; 130(6):1216–23.
5. Georghiou GP, Porat E, Fuks A, et al. Video-assisted pericardial fenestration for effusions after cardiac surgery. Asian Cardiovasc Thorac Ann 2009;17(5):480–2.
6. Pepi M, Muratori M, Barbier P, et al. Pericardial effusion after cardiac surgery: incidence, site, size, and haemodynamic consequences. Br Heart J 1994;72:327–31.
7. Al-Dadah AS, Guthrie TJ, Pasque MK, et al. Clinical course and predictors of pericardial effusion following cardiac transplantation. Transplant Proc 2007;39: 1589–92.
8. Alpert MA, Ravenscraft MD. Pericardial involvement in end-stage renal disease. Am J Med Sci 2003;325(4):228–36.
9. Leehey DJ, Daugirdas JT, Popli S, et al. Predicting need for surgical drainage of pericardial effusion in patients with end-stage renal disease. Int J Artif Organs 1989;12:618–25.

10. Spodick DH. Acute cardiac tamponade. N Engl J Med 2003;349:684–90.
11. Meltser H, Kalaria VG. Cardiac tamponade. Catheter Cardiovasc Interv 2005;64: 245–55.
12. Hoit BD. Cardiac tamponade. Available at: http://www.uptodate.com. Accessed May 1, 2009.
13. Goldberger AL. Electrocardiogram in pericarditis and pericardial tamponade. Available at: http://www.uptodate.com. Accessed September 30, 2009.
14. Lake CL. Anesthesia and pericardial disease. Anesth Analg 1983;62:431–43.
15. Wann S, Passen E. Echocardiography in pericardial disease. J Am Soc Echocardiogr 2008;21(1):7–13.
16. Seferovic PM, Ristic AD, Imazio M, et al. Management strategies in pericardial emergencies. Herz 2006;31(9):891–900.
17. Moores DW, Dziuban SW Jr. Pericardial drainage procedures. Chest Surg Clin N Am 1995;5(2):359–73.
18. Lui H, Chang C, Lin PJ, et al. Thoracoscopic management of effusive pericardial disease: indications and technique. Ann Thorac Surg 1994;58:1695–7.
19. Olsen PS, Sorensen C, Andersen HO. Surgical treatment of large pericardial effusions. Eur J Cardiothorac Surg 1991;5:430–2.
20. Olson JE, Ryan MB, Blumenstock DA. Eleven years' experience with pericardial-peritoneal window in the management of malignant and benign pericardial effusions. Ann Surg Oncol 1995;2(2):165–9.
21. Aye T, Miline B. Ketamine anesthesia for pericardial window in a patient with pericardial tamponade and severe COPD. Can J Anaesth 2002;49(3):283–6.
22. Van Tright P, Douglas J, Smith PK, et al. A prospective trial of subxiphoid pericardiotomy in the diagnosis and treatment of large pericardial effusion. Ann Surg 1993;218(6):777–82.
23. Vassilopoulos PP, Nikolaidis K, Filopoulos E, et al. Subxiphoidal pericardial 'window' in the management of malignant pericardial effusion. Eur J Surg Oncol 1995;21:545–7.
24. Sinzobahamvya N. Results of subxiphoid pericardiostomy in pericardial effusion. Acta Chir Belg 1988;88:175–8.
25. Bernal JM, Afonso L, Pradhan J, et al. Acute pulmonary edema following pericardiocentesis for cardiac tamponade. Can J Cardiol 2007;23(14):1155–6.
26. Vandyke WH Jr, Cure J, Chakko CS, et al. Pulmonary edema after pericardiocentesis for cardiac tamponade. N Engl J Med 1983;309:595–6.
27. Chamoun A, Cenz R, Mager A, et al. Acute left ventricular failure after large volume pericardiocentesis. Clin Cardiol 2003;26:588–90.
28. Hamaya Y, Dohi S, Ueda N, et al. Severe circulatory collapse immediately after pericardiocentesis in a patient with chronic cardiac tamponade. Anesth Analg 1993;77:1278–81.
29. Karamichalis JM, Gursky A, Valaulikar G, et al. Acute pulmonary edema after pericardial drainage for cardiac tamponade. Ann Thorac Surg 2009;88(2):675–7.
30. Downey RJ, Bessler M, Weissman C. Acute pulmonary edema following pericardiocentesis for chronic cardiac tamponade secondary to trauma. Crit Care Med 1991;19(10):1323–5.
31. Brooker RF, Testa LD, Butterworth J, et al. Diagnosis and management of acute hypoxemia after drainage of massive pericardial effusion. J Cardiothorac Vasc Anesth 1998;12(1):69–71.
32. Webster JA, Self DD. Anesthesia for pericardial window in a pregnant patient with cardiac tamponade and mediastinal mass. Can J Anaesth 2003;50(8):815–8.

Anesthetic Concerns in Trauma Victims Requiring Operative Intervention: The Patient Too Sick to Anesthetize

Maureen McCunn, MD, MIPP, FCCM*, Emily K.B. Gordon, MD, Thomas H. Scott, MD

KEYWORDS

- Multiple trauma • Injury • Shock • Resuscitation
- Massive transfusion • Damage control • Extracorporeal

Trauma is the third leading cause of death overall in the United States, and the leading cause of death among those aged 1 to 44 years. Nearly 30% of years of potential life lost before age 65 results from traumatic injury, the largest contribution of any cause of death and nearly twice that of the next leading cause, cancer.[1] Globally, the World Health Organization projects a 40% increase in global deaths caused by injury between 2002 and 2030.[2] As this burden of injury increases, anesthesiology practitioners will be challenged with the operative case management of this disease.

Case study. You are the anesthesiologist caring for an obese 66-year-old man who was involved in a motor vehicle crash; he was not wearing a seat belt. The patient presents to the operating room (OR) for emergency exploratory laparotomy. Blood pressure (BP) 83/P, heart rate 128, So_2 94% on 1.0 Fio_2 per endotracheal tube, Glasgow Coma Scale 5T, temperature 35.2°C. The patient has ecchymoses over the right face, contusions over the sternum, a flail chest, distended abdomen, and a pelvic binder in place. Crystalloids are infusing through a 14G peripheral intravenous line and the first unit of packed red blood cells (PRBC) is hanging. What are your management priorities and the interventions that you can provide to improve this patient's outcome?

Department of Anesthesiology and Critical Care, University of Pennsylvania School of Medicine, Dulles 6, 3400 Spruce Street, Philadelphia, PA 19104, USA
* Corresponding author.
E-mail address: mccunnm@uphs.upenn.edu

Anesthesiology Clin 28 (2010) 97–116
doi:10.1016/j.anclin.2010.01.004   **anesthesiology.theclinics.com**

CARDIAC TRAUMA

Cardiac trauma may complicate anesthetic management of patients following injury, particularly in the patient with preexisting comorbidities on multiple medications. Traditional markers of myocardial ischemia such as electrocardiogram (ECG) changes and increased enzyme levels may be misleading in the patient who has sustained a massive energy transfer to their thorax from trauma. Blunt thoracic trauma constitutes 25% of all trauma mortalities,[3] and can have a vast range of clinical presentations. Hemodynamic instability raises a high index of suspicion for blunt myocardial injury (BMI), previously referred to as cardiac contusion, pericardial tamponade, blunt thoracic aortic injury, and myocardial infarction. Cardiac and thoracic vasculature must be evaluated during the initial trauma work-up.

Blunt traumatic aortic injury (TAI) is typically seen in rapid deceleration and crush injuries. Approximately 85% of these patients die at the scene,[4] often from concomitant nonsurvivable injuries. For those who reach the hospital, the severity of thoracic skeletal injury often may not correlate with the severity of aortic injury. TAI can be seen after a fall, and side impact in a motor vehicle crash is a major risk factor, both of which highlight the mechanism of injury: deceleration to the entire body, not just a direct blow to the chest. Despite optimal medical care, approximately 50% of patients who make it to the hospital die in the first 24 hours of hospitalization,[5] often as a result of associated trauma. The classic clinical signs and symptoms of aortic injury are chest pain, pseudocoarctation, aortic insufficiency murmur, and sternal fractures; patients may be asymptomatic from TAI and the diagnosis is made during radiologic evaluation. A patient who arrives in the emergency department (ED) after sustaining blunt thoracic trauma should have an ECG to evaluate for dysrhythmia or ECG changes. If a patient has no ECG changes on arrival then there is a lower likelihood of any cardiac injury.[6,7] If there are ECG changes, further evaluation is warranted. This evaluation should include cardiac markers (cardiac troponin T and I), with consideration of transesophageal or transthoracic echocardiography (TEE or TTE). TEE is more sensitive and specific than TTE in the detection of BMI, valvular injury, and aortic injury.[7] Pharmacologic management is aimed toward blood pressure and heart rate control, and hemodynamic stability may be best achieved with high-dose narcotic and β blockade, particularly if the patient has hemorrhage as a result of associated injuries.

Widening of the mediastinum on the chest radiograph is nonspecific and may frequently not be present in cases of severe aortic trauma. Although aortography is still held by many to be the gold standard, advancements in computed tomography angiography (CTA) have allowed it to largely replace older techniques in preoperative evaluation.[8] The other advantage of CTA is its ability to identify other significant diagnoses (eg, blunt cerebrovascular injury).

In the last 10 years endovascular stent grafting has become widely used to treat blunt thoracic aortic injury. No prospective, randomized, controlled clinical trials have yet compared stent graft placement with open repair. Meta-analyses of retrospective studies have suggested better outcomes from stent graft placement compared with open repair. Most of these studies show that mortality, paraplegia, and stroke occur less often with delayed endovascular repair.[9–11] Others have found no decrease in mortality but a decrease in neurologic injury.[12] Although there are insufficient long-term outcome data, it does seem that endovascular repair is a reasonable and effective treatment of blunt thoracic aortic injury.

Transient left ventricular apical ballooning, also known as Tako Tsubo syndrome, is a reversible cardiomyopathy described in patients with high exposure to catecholamine. The description of this syndrome, leading to refractory hypotension associated with multiple trauma,[13] highlights an important fact: many patients who have myocardial insufficiency following injury will have complete recovery of cardiac function with resolution of traumatic illness.

There is no standard anesthetic management schema for cardiac trauma; some disease presentations have significantly different management strategies than nontrauma presentations (eg, systolic anterior motion). A pericardial window is often critical in the evaluation of a hemodynamically stable patient who is suspected of having a cardiac injury.[14] A wide variety of cardiac injuries that can occur secondary to trauma are outlined in **Table 1**.

PULMONARY TRAUMA

The trauma patient with underlying lung disease presents with 2 classes of pulmonary complications: those attributable to the traumatic injury per se, and those caused by underlying medical comorbidities that are exacerbated by the traumatic insult. Older patients with preexisting pulmonary disease are at greater risk of perioperative and postoperative pulmonary complications than young patients with healthy lungs.[30] Moreover, perioperative lung complications may be as prevalent and as predictive of mortality as perioperative cardiac complications.[31,32] There is little evidence to suggest that interventions taken by an anesthesiologist during the perioperative period might reduce postoperative pulmonary complications in patients with traumatic injury.[32] This section focuses on the 2 most common and life-threatening pulmonary problems faced by anesthesiologists during acute trauma: inability to oxygenate and inability to ventilate (**Table 2**).

Cannot Oxygenate: Hypoxia

In the intubated trauma patient receiving a high Fio_2, hypoxia results from a high fraction of pulmonary blood flow failing to perfuse ventilated portions of the lungs before reentering the systemic circulation. Although an increased shunt fraction is most commonly caused by intrapulmonary pathology, it can also be intracardiac and this may only become physiologically significant after another insult causes higher pulmonary artery pressures (ie, fat embolism syndrome (FES), pulmonary embolism (PE), acute lung injury (ALI), and aspiration pneumonitis).

Blunt chest trauma can result in pulmonary contusions and flail chest. Development of pulmonary contusions is independently associated with development of acute lung injury/acute respiratory distress syndrome (ALI/ARDS), pneumonia, and death.[33] Increasing age and medical comorbidities (congestive heart failure, cirrhosis, renal dysfunction, and others) are also independently associated with sepsis and death in thoracic trauma with rib fractures.[34] Even small pulmonary contusions can, within 24 hours, create an inflammatory cascade leading to increased pulmonary capillary permeability, decreased surfactant production, alveolar collapse, and predisposition to sepsis by inhibiting macrophage and lymphocyte immune function.[35] Moreover, clinically significant pulmonary contusions are often missed on initial chest radiography. Computed tomography (CT) of the chest is the gold standard for diagnosis. Thus, management of patients with pulmonary contusions should focus on, in addition to maintaining oxygenation, avoiding a second assault on the lungs such as aspiration, fat embolism, sepsis, or ventilator-induced lung injury. Intraoperative management strategies should include open-lung pressure-limited ventilation if hemodynamically tolerated and minimizing inspired Fio_2 in the absence of shock.[36]

Flail chest is defined as at least 2 ribs broken in 2 places causing an invagination of the chest wall with each attempt at respiration. Like pulmonary contusions, flail chest

Table 1
Traumatic cardiac injuries, typical presentation, diagnostic evaluation and treatment strategies

Injury	Diagnosis	Presentation	Treatment
Blunt myocardial injury[6,7]	Typically seen following blunt chest trauma. Presentation ranges from asymptomatic to cardiac rupture	ECG changes, wall motion abnormalities on TTE/TEE	Monitor telemetry and CE; increased risk of arrhythmia, late rupture, aneurysm formation, CHF and intracavitary thrombus
Traumatic VSD[15,16]	Typically seen after unrestrained MVC; panholosystolic murmur at left lower sternal border with precordial thrill. Rare complication of trauma and can be present with no symptoms or can result in heart failure	TTE or TEE; may have increase in cardiac enzymes (although this is an overly sensitive marker as high-energy transfer from trauma may also cause increase in enzymes). ECG changes are more predictive	Immediate or delayed surgical treatment dependent on clinical symptoms and size of defect. Multiple case studies of traumatic VSDs that were not repaired in patients who have remained healthy
Cardiac foreign bodies[17]	Traumatic versus iagtrogenic. Ranges from symptom free to cardiac tamponade or hemorrhagic shock	Chest radiograph, CT scan, echocardiography (immediate or delayed)	Surgery versus conservative treatment depending on patient's symptoms, position of object, and associated risks of embolization
Papillary muscle/ chordae tendinae rupture[18,19]	No symptoms to acute cardiogenic shock; holosystolic murmur at the apex radiating to axilla. Most common injury is to mitral valve	TTE or TEE	Surgical intervention based on hemodynamic stability and other associated injuries; mitral valve replacement versus subvalvular repair
Systolic anterior motion[20,21]	Typically seen in association with hypovolemia or anesthesia-mediated vasodilatation hypotension	Diagnosed with echocardiography; can be difficult to diagnose. Patient will either be predisposed or this will be a preinjury disease; not caused by trauma per se	Phenylephrine and fluid resuscitation; possible use of β-blockers in those with relative reductions in preload
Penetrating cardiac injury[22,23]	Pericardial tamponade to hemorrhagic shock depending on whether the pericardium is violated	FAST scan in ED has high sensitivity and specificity; pericardial window is the gold standard to confirm cardiac injury	Pericardial window, thoracotomy or median sternotomy

Cardiac tamponade[24]	Muffled heart tones, pulsus paradoxus, increased CVP, bulging neck veins, signs of shock	FAST scan in ED has high sensitivity and specificity	Delay induction of anesthesia if possible until surgeon in OR to assume direct control of the cardiac injury if hemodynamic instability
Blunt cardiac rupture or rupture of major vessels[25-28]	Varies, but typically with hypotension and hemorrhagic shock; may or may not have tamponade symptoms	High degree of suspicion is necessary; FAST, TTE or TEE	Possible need for emergency thoracotomy; immediate OR intervention
Blunt aortic injury[9-12,26,29]	Typically seen after rapid deceleration injuries. Presentation ranges from asymptomatic to hemodynamic instability	Injury identified by CTA or echocardiogram	Immediate versus delayed surgical repair. Endovascular stent placement versus primary repair

Signs and symptoms may be difficult to assess in patients with multiple injuries in a noisy/chaotic trauma bay.

Abbreviations: CE, cardiac enzymes; CHF, chronic heart failure; CT, computed tomography; CTA, computed tomographic angiography; CVP, central venous pressure; ECG, electrocardiogram; FAST, focused abdominal sonography for trauma; MVC, motor vehicle crash; TTE/TEE, transthoracic/transesophageal echocardiography; VSD, ventricular septal defect.

can lead to respiratory failure, from splinting because of chest wall pain. Adequate analgesia and effective pulmonary toilet are essential management goals. However, opiates, the mainstay of analgesia in most trauma and general surgery patients, depress the central respiratory drive, making them a suboptimal choice in the setting of flail chest. Neuraxial analgesia (epidural catheters or intercostal nerve blocks) in the setting of flail chest can be helpful, preventing intubation, and reducing duration of mechanical ventilation and time to discharge from the intensive care unit (ICU), and the incidence of nosocomial pneumonia.[37,38]

FES is an under-recognized pulmonary complication. FES has variable clinical definitions and a wide range of reported clinical incidence (0.25%–35%) in acute trauma.[39] Fat particles are identified in the pulmonary arteries in 90% of patients with skeletal trauma.[39] Major diagnostic criteria include a petechial rash, altered mental status, and respiratory insufficiency. Minor nonspecific signs include tachypnea, tachycardia, hypoxia, hypercapnea, and infiltrates on chest radiography. Severity of presentation can be fulminant or subacute and occurs 12–24 hours after injury or with surgical manipulation of long-bone fractures. Other risk factors include delayed stabilization of long-bone or pelvic fractures, male gender, age 10 to 40 years, multiple long-bone fractures, and surgical internal fixation of long-bone fractures with intramedullary reaming.[40] Because the signs and symptoms of FES are nonspecific and the treatment of FES is supportive, preventing FES and maintaining a high index of suspicion for FES is critical. Prompt fixation of pelvic and long-bone fractures may be the most effective means of avoiding FES.[41,42] If FES is present, or if there is a high suspicion of FES, manipulating long bones for definitive internal fixation may exacerbate

Table 2
Differential diagnosis and treatment of pulmonary complications of traumatic injury

	Cannot Ventilate	Cannot Oxygenate
Abnormality	High peak, high plateau pressures	Increased intrapulmonary shunt fraction
Nontraumatic causes	Auto-PEEP; CHF flare; morbid obesity; Trendelenburg position; abdominal compartment syndrome; pleural effusion	Preexisting obstructive or parenchymal lung disease (asthma, COPD); pulmonary fibrosis; bronchiectasis; pulmonary edema; aspiration pneumonitis; pulmonary embolism; TRALI
Traumatic causes	Tension pneumothorax; pulmonary contusion; ARDS (may present acutely following pulmonary contusion, aspiration or massive transfusion); gastrothorax; hemothorax	Pulmonary contusions; ARDS; pulmonary laceration; fat emboli syndrome (with long-bone fractures or massive soft tissue injury); aspiration; TRALI
Management options	• Needle decompression and tube thoracosomy if breath sounds absent and tension physiology present • Consider Auto-PEEP • Try disconnecting patient from the ventilator temporarily, allowing any trapped gas to escape • If BP and plateau pressures improve, auto-PEEP is likely present and high peak flows should be tolerated provided that plateau pressures can be kept less than 35 cm H_2O • Prolong the inspiratory/expiratory ratio to ensure that the flow reaches zero at end expiration • May require tolerating hypercapnea • Review preoperative CT scan chest, consider intraoperative ultrasound/TTE/TEE • Intraoperative bronchoscopy • Check circuit and endotracheal tube patency • Suction airways • Endotracheal bronchodilators • Consider PE or fat embolism	• Examine patient for evidence of reversible causes • Wheezing (obstructive lung disease, PE/fat emboli, CHF) • Trial of bronchodilators and/or dieresis • Moderate intraoperative fluids • Recruitment maneuvers, PEEP (prevent derecruitment) • Consider avoiding manipulation and/or intramedullary reaming of long bones • Extracorporeal support

Abbreviations: COPD, chronic obstructive pulmonary disease; PEEP, positive end-expiratory pressure.

FES, causing clinical deterioration. Treatment options in this scenario include external fixation and avoiding definitive intramedullary internal fixation until clinical signs of FES have stabilized.[43] Rapidly progressive hypoxemia and worsening pulmonary compliance should alert the anesthesiologist to the possibility of FES, which can also occur with soft tissue injury (**Fig. 1**). A differential diagnosis should include other traumatic

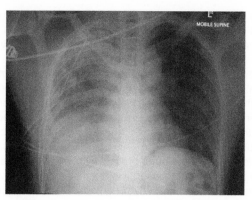

Fig. 1. Blunt thoracic trauma. Patient has right hemothorax, pneumothorax and pulmonary contusion. Hypoxia, high peak inspiratory pressure, and myocardial dysfunction are present.

causes such as pneumothorax, pulmonary contusion, severe aspiration, and volume overload from massive resuscitation.

Transfusion-related acute lung injury (TRALI) is noncardiogenic pulmonary edema resulting from immune reactivity of certain leukocyte antibodies a few hours after transfusion. Signs and symptoms appear 1 to 2 hours after transfusion and peak within 6 hours. Hypoxia, fever, dyspnea, and even fluid in the endotracheal tube may occur. There is no specific therapy other than stopping transfusion and instituting critical care supportive measures. Most patients recover in 96 hours, although TRALI is 1 of the top 3 most common causes of transfusion-related deaths.[44–46]

Cannot Ventilate: High Ventilator Pressures

Increased peak pressures and normal plateau pressures often reflect large airway obstruction from various causes; a differential diagnosis following trauma includes blood, food particles, and foreign bodies. Conversely, increased peak pressures and plateau pressures can reflect decreased pulmonary, diaphragmatic, and/or chest wall compliance (see **Table 2**). Worsening compliance is an ominous situation as it may be associated with hypoxia.

To differentiate between high peak and high plateau pressure, blow a fixed volume of air into the ventilator under high flows, with high-pressure cut-offs such that the entire tidal volume can be delivered and the inspiratory flow reaches zero before expiration. The end-inspiratory pressure at a zero flow rate is the plateau pressure, or the inspiratory pressure at the level of the alveoli. The peak pressure is simply the peak pressure generated by a given tidal volume at a given flow rate and reflects bronchial, large airway, or endotracheal tube resistance more so than plateau pressure. The peak pressure will be higher with smaller-size endotracheal tubes, or those partially occluded with blood, pulmonary debris, or secretions.

Fig. 1 is a chest radiograph of a patient with a constellation of thoracic injuries that may lead to cardiopulmonary insufficiency and progress to cardiac and respiratory collapse. When mechanical ventilation fails to achieve adequate oxygenation and/or carbon dioxide (CO_2) exchange, extracorporeal support can be a life-saving treatment option following trauma (see later discussion).

NEUROLOGIC INJURIES

Traumatic brain injury (TBI) and hemorrhagic shock are the 2 leading causes of death from trauma. Central nervous system injury is the most common cause of civilian deaths from injury, but hemorrhage and resultant multiple organ system failure account for almost half of all deaths and almost all of the deaths that are available for secondary prevention.[47] It is not uncommon to see these devastating diseases concurrently.

Severe TBI is known to be 1 of the most important prognostic factors in patients with trauma, with mortality in 1 series of patients with head injures about 3 times higher than in patients without relevant TBI (22.1% vs 7.3%).[48] The reasons are likely multifactorial, including interplay between the neuroendocrine system and the injured brain. A catecholamine surge occurs after TBI[49–51] that may manifest as acute hemodynamic instability and respiratory failure in the OR. Subendocardial ischemia may lead to biventricular heart failure, even in young previously healthy patients. Acute cardiopulmonary failure may be exacerbated when treated with exogenous vasoactive agents, perpetuating a cycle of ischemia. Rapidly progressive cardiopulmonary collapse with increased intracranial pressure (ICP), resulting from severe TBI, can be successfully treated with extracorporeal life support.[52,53] A 16-year-old and a 20-year-old with TBI after blunt trauma each developed cardiac failure (ejection fraction by echocardiography 20%, and 10%, respectively), ARDS, and multiorgan failure. Anticoagulation was not used for 24 hours in the 16-year-old (total extracorporeal life support [ECLS] time 4 days) and not at all in the 20-year-old patient (total ECLS time 49 hours). Both patients had full neurologic recovery.

β blockade has been shown to be protective in human studies in patients with brain injuries. Retrospective database reviews have shown neurologic improvement and a survival advantage associated with β blockade following TBI.[54–56] The largest series to date reported a significant decrease in mortality for patients with severe TBI (50% for those exposed to β blockade vs 70% for those who were not). On subgroup analysis, elderly patients with severe injury had a mortality of 28% on β-blockers compared with 60% when they did not receive them ($P = .001$).[54] Intraoperative initiation of β blockade in the acute management of patients with TBI has not been studied.

Non-neurologic organ dysfunction is common in patients with severe TBI and is independently associated with worse outcome.[57,58] Of 209 consecutive patients with TBI, 89% developed dysfunction of at least 1 non-neurologic organ system. Respiratory failure was the most common, followed by cardiovascular failure. Failure of the coagulation and renal systems was also seen.[57]

In the absence of ICP and cerebral oxygenation monitoring, the goals to achieve optimal cerebral perfusion and oxygenation are systolic blood pressure >90 mm Hg and Pao_2 >60 (So_2 >90%). Management of elevated ICP intraoperatively may be accomplished with mannitol (0.25–1 g/kg) with particular attention to avoidance of hypovolemia (systolic BP >90 mm Hg) and maintenance of intravascular volume status, or hypertonic saline (HTS). The use of HTS for ICP control developed from studies on small volume resuscitation in multitrauma patients in hemorrhagic shock. The subgroup with TBI showed the greatest survival benefit, while preserving or even improving hemodynamic parameters.[59] Although the use of mannitol has become commonplace, most of the discussion in the guidelines surrounds the increasing evidence for effectiveness and safety of HTS in treating increased ICP. Current research is ongoing.

Although robust data are lacking, the American Association of Neurologic Surgeons Guidelines for the Management of Acute Cervical Spine and Spinal Cord Injuries suggest maintenance of mean arterial pressure 85 to 90 mm Hg for the first 7 days following acute spinal cord injury to improve spinal cord perfusion.[60] Maintenance of cerebral and spinal cord perfusion pressures can be a challenge in patients with exsanguinating hemorrhage, in those with acute cardiorespiratory failure as a result of their neurologic injury, or in patients with neurogenic shock. Vasoactive agents that increase peripheral resistance and concomitantly add inotropic support may be advantageous.

EXSANGUINATION/COAGULATION ABNORMALITIES

Bleeding is the most frequent cause of preventable death after severe injury. Penetrating injury to solid organs or major vasculature, and blunt trauma resulting in high-grade pelvic fractures, significant solid organ lacerations, or massive tissue destruction may lead to exsanguination (**Fig. 2**). Maintaining a low mean arterial blood pressure (controlled hypotension) decreases mortality following penetrating trauma[61] and is safe following blunt trauma.[62] The Advanced Trauma Life Support Course (ATLS) now includes a far more extensive discussion on the importance of balancing the concept of limited resuscitation with excessive early crystalloid administration that may dilute blood, dislodge clot, and increase hemorrhage. A recent retrospective review did not show a difference in mortality in patients with penetrating truncal injury who received limited crystalloid resuscitation in the field[63]; larger randomized prospective trials are still needed.[64] The American Society of Anesthesiologists has published guidelines for blood transfusion and adjuvant therapies.[44] Unfortunately for the trauma patient who requires acute operative intervention, there is rarely time for preoperative assessment of possible bleeding abnormalities. The American Society of Anesthesiologists recommends transfusion to maintain hemoglobin level >6 g/dL, prothrombin time (PT) greater than 1.5 times normal or international normalized ratio greater than 2.0, an activated partial prothrombin time greater than 2 times normal, platelets 50,000 cells/mm^3, and fibrinogen <80 mg/dL as a guide to therapy, but reliance on laboratory values should not delay product infusion in a patient with acute traumatic exsanguination. Classic resuscitation strategies have been called into question by recent findings.[65]

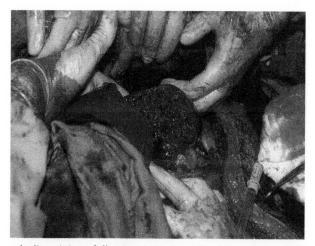

Fig. 2. High-grade liver injury following intraoperative hemorrhage control. Controlled under-resuscitation (delayed resuscitation), with mean arterial pressure of 50 to 60 mm Hg may decrease blood loss. This management strategy is challenging in a patient with traumatic brain or spinal cord injury, and in those with known preexisting cardiac or vascular disease.

At the time of arrival at the emergency department, approximately 25% of trauma patients have a detectable coagulopathy that is associated with poor outcome, and increased PT and partial thromboplastin time are independent predictors of mortality.[66,67] **Fig. 3** shows the type of injury that may lead to coagulopathy; massive resuscitation of these patients increases the risk of pulmonary and cardiac insufficiency. There is a positive correlation with injury severity score and coagulopathy, but dilution of clotting factors through infusion of intravenous fluids is not the only mechanism.[66] Coagulopathy associated with traumatic injury is the result of multiple independent but interacting mechanisms: early coagulopathy is driven by shock and requires thrombin generation from tissue injury as an initiator; initiation of coagulation occurs with activation of anticoagulant and fibrinolytic pathways. This acute coagulopathy of trauma-shock (ACoTS) is altered by subsequent events and medical therapies, including acidemia, hypothermia, and dilution. ACoTS should be considered distinct from disseminated intravascular coagulation as described in other conditions.[68,69]

The concept of damage control resuscitation attempts to address early coagulopathy and advocates transfusing earlier and with increased amounts of plasma and platelets along with the first units of red blood cells, while simultaneously minimizing crystalloid use in patients who are predicted to require a massive transfusion (MT). Patients who require MT represent a small percentage of admissions (3%), yet have a 30% to 60% mortality.[70,71] A recent review of records of 467 MT civilian trauma patients transported from the scene to 16 level 1 trauma centers between July 2005 and June 2006 correlated transfusion ratios with mortality.[72] The plasma/RBC ratio ranged from 0 to 2.89 (mean ± SD 0.56 ± 0.35) and the platelets/RBC ratio ranged from 0 to 2.5 (0.55 ± 0.50). Plasma/RBC and platelet/RBC ratios and injury severity score were predictors of death at 6 hours, 24 hours, and 30 days in multivariate logistic models. Thirty-day survival was increased in patients with high plasma/RBC ratio (>1:2) relative to those with low plasma/RBC ratio (≤1:2) (low 40.4% vs high 59.6%, $P<.01$). Similarly, 30-day survival was increased in patients with high platelet/RBC ratio (>1:2) relative to those with low platelet/RBC ratio (≤1:2) (low

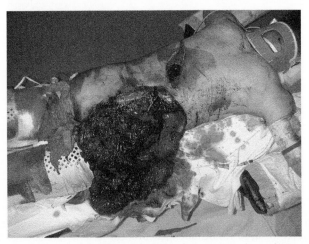

Fig. 3. Massive right gluteal degloving injury following motorcycle crash. Coagulopathy and cardiopulmonary dysfunction are present. (Patient is in the prone position on the OR table, head to the right and lower extremities on the left.)

40.1% vs high 59.9%, $P<.01$). In patients with combat-related trauma requiring MT, the transfusion of an increased fibrinogen/RBC ratio was independently associated with improved survival to hospital discharge, primarily by decreasing the number of deaths from hemorrhage.[73] A retrospective chart review of 252 patients at a US Army combat support hospital who received MT (>10 units of RBCs in 24 hours) used the amount of fibrinogen within each blood product to calculate the fibrinogen/RBC (F/R) ratio transfused for each patient. The mean (SD) F/R ratios transfused for the low and high groups were 0.1 g/unit ($\pm$ 0.06), and 0.48 g/unit ($\pm$ 0.2), respectively ($P<.001$). Mortality was 52% and 24% in the low and high F/R ratio groups respectively ($P<.001$). Clinicians can meet this requirement by transfusing 1 unit of FFP for every 2 units of red cells, or by transfusing one 10-unit bag of cryoprecipitate for every 10 units of red cells. High concentrations of fibrinogen are available not only from cryoprecipitate but also from plasma-derived fibrinogen concentrates. Fibrinogen is also now being produced using recombinant techniques and is available in a lyophilized powder form (Pharming Group, Leiden, The Netherlands).

MT protocols in the United States are now incorporating early use of balanced resuscitation.[74,75] The optimal ratio of blood products has not yet been determined, although many agree that an FFP/PRBC transfusion ratio greater than 1:1.5 is best.[76] In patients requiring more than 8 units of blood after serious blunt injury, an FFP/PRBC transfusion ratio greater than 1:1.5 was associated with a significantly lower risk of mortality but a higher risk of acute respiratory distress syndrome. However, in a recent review of humans who received aggressive factor replacement, data collected on 806 consecutive trauma patients admitted to the intensive care unit for 2 years showed no significant difference in outcome when comparing patients who had a 1:1 PRBC/FFP ratio with those who did not receive any FFP.[77] Patients were stratified by PRBC/FFP transfusion ratio in the first 24 hours. Analyzing these patients by stepwise regression controlling for all significant variables, the PRBC/FFP ratio did not predict intensive care unit days, hospital days, or mortality even in patients who received MT ($\geq$10 U). In a more recent study, FFP was associated with higher incidence of multiple organ failure and ARDS.[78] Data were obtained from a multicenter prospective cohort study evaluating clinical outcomes in bluntly injured adults with hemorrhagic shock who required blood transfusion. Patients with isolated TBI and those not surviving beyond 48 hours were excluded. Cox proportional hazard regression models were used to estimate the outcome risks (per unit) associated with plasma-rich transfusion requirements during the initial 24 hours after injury after controlling for important confounders. There was no association with plasma-rich transfusion components and mortality or nosocomial infection. However, for every unit given, FFP was independently associated with a 2.1% and 2.5% increased risk of multiorgan failure and ARDS, respectively. Cryoprecipitate was associated with a 4.4% decreased risk of multiorgan failure (per unit), and platelets were not associated with any of the outcomes examined. When early deaths (within 48 hours) were included in the model, FFP was associated with a 2.9% decreased risk of mortality per unit transfused. Conflicting data such as that presented here, in addition to mounting evidence that transfusion of stored blood increases mortality,[79] organ dysfunction,[80] nosocomial infections[81] and resource use,[82] challenge the acute care provider to make appropriate resuscitation decisions.

Several investigators have recently described the proinflammatory characteristics of crystalloid infusion[83–86]; others have described decreased abdominal compartment syndrome and death[87] or increased ventilator and ICU-free days[88] simply by limiting the amount of crystalloid infused early after admission. Plasma has been shown to be less inflammatory than artificial colloid, albumin, or lactated Ringer solution in an animal study of hemorrhagic shock.[85]

Adjuvant therapies to address coagulopathy include topical hemostatic dressings,[89,90] widely used in the military,[91,92] and recombinant factor VIIa.[93,94] Often cited as a concern in the use of rFVIIa, the cost of the drug has limited its use in many centers. It would seem that the optimal dose of rFVIIa is still not known. Although early studies used doses of 100–200 µg/kg after more than 10 units of PRBC,[95,96] more recent data suggest earlier administration[96] and a lower dose of VIIa (1.2 mg) is not only effective for coagulopathy[97] but is also more cost-effective than plasma, and decreases the number of blood products transfused.[96,98,99] In a 5-year retrospective chart review of coagulopathic patients with TBI, total mean charges and costs, in addition to hospital length of stay, days of mechanical ventilation, and plasma transfused, were significantly lower in the group that received rFVIIa compared with those that did not ($US 77,907 vs $108,900). There was no difference in thromboembolic complications between the groups. In another retrospective review, factor VIIa also decreased time to neurosurgical intervention (ICP monitor or craniotomy), number of units of plasma transfused, and was associated with lower mortality (33.3% in the rFVIIa group and 52.9% in controls; $P = .24$) without a difference in thromboembolic rates.[97] Administration of rVIIa should not be seen as a rescue therapy, and may be less effective when administered late in resuscitation efforts.[95] Earlier use is associated with lower rates of total blood products transfused.[94]

ORTHOPEDIC INJURIES

There is extensive debate in the trauma literature regarding timing of fraction fixation (early vs delayed)[100] and type of fixation (stabilizing vs definitive),[43,101] particularly if concurrent traumatic brain or chest injury exists.[102] Without adequate fixation, the patient cannot be mobilized; this can result in dysfunction of multiple organ systems.[103] However, overly aggressive orthopedic fixation within 24 hours of admission in multitrauma patients seems to be associated with an increased complication rate.[104] This has led to an approach that takes into account an individual patients' clinical condition (blood pressure, coagulation status, temperature, severity of injury) to guide treatment, and includes a discussion between the trauma and orthopedic surgeons, anesthesiologist, and consulting services (eg, neurosurgery).[103] Patients known to be at higher risk of perioperative complications include injury severity score greater than 40, multiple injuries in association with thoracic, abdominal or pelvic injury + shock (blood pressure <90 mm Hg), radiographic evidence of pulmonary contusion, temperature less than 35°C, and moderate-severe brain injury.[103] Pelvic fractures can be life-threatening and often require acute operative intervention for fixation or packing.[105,106] Surgery should not be delayed and damage control resuscitation may include angiographic embolization.

EXTRACORPOREAL LIFE SUPPORT

The various uses of ECLS following trauma are well known.[107–113] In addition to the cases cited earlier for ECLS following TBI, recent reports continue to illustrate the safe use of ECLS following traumatic injury. A case series by Huang and colleagues,[114] from March 2004 to October 2007, reports on 9 patients with posttraumatic ARDS who had failed conventional therapies including surgical interventions. Median time interval from trauma to ECLS was 33 hours (range 4–383 hours) and median duration of ECLS was 145 hours (range 68–456 hours). Six patients (66.7%) received additional surgeries while on ECLS; 7 patients (77.8%) were weaned and discharged. The traumas included grade 3 or 4 liver lacerations, a grade 3 spleen laceration, and TBI. Clinicians in Germany have also had recent success with venoarterial extracorporeal membrane oxygenation in treating a series of patients with ARDS following severe chest injury in multitrauma patients.[115] One of the most exciting advances to be published recently is the use of a pumpless extracorporeal circuit, which is inherently simple, efficient, and allows for easier intrahospital and interhospital patient transport, and has the potential to allow for international transport,[116] as may be necessary to evacuate soldiers from conflict zones. The review by Flörchinger and colleagues[116] describes 10 years of experience with pumpless extracorporeal lung assist (PECLA) used in 159 patients (age range 7–78 years). Weaning was successful in 52.2% and overall survival to hospital discharge was 33.1% of patients after a mean PECLA support of 8.5 ± 6.3 days. The best outcomes were obtained in patients after trauma (n = 37).

COEXISTING DISEASES AND OUTCOME FOLLOWING TRAUMA

Increasing age has been associated with higher mortality following trauma[117,118] but until recently the role of concomitant preinjury diseases that are common with advancing age was not clear. Analysis of records of 11,142 trauma patients for a 5-year period from the trauma registry of the German Society for Trauma Surgery revealed preexisting medical conditions in 34.4% of patients.[119] Logistic regression for age-adjusted analysis showed the following preexisting conditions to be associated with increased mortality: heart disease, hepatitis/liver cirrhosis, carcinoma, obesity, and peripheral arterial occlusive disease. Previous studies have shown obesity (body mass index [BMI, calculated as weight in kilograms divided by the square of height in meters] >30 kg/m^2),[120–122] and liver disease[123–125] (independent of coagulation disturbances) to be independent risk factors for mortality. However, worse outcomes in geriatric trauma patients cannot be caused by preexisting disease solely, as the results from the German Trauma Registry confirm the independent predictive value of age in multivariable analysis. Changes in posttraumatic immune response with subsequent multiorgan failure may also be responsible for high mortality in geriatric patients.[117,126]

Table 3
Selected examples of intraoperative management of trauma-related diagnoses that vary from traditional nontrauma causes of life-threatening disorders (see text for discussion)

Medical Condition	Traditional Treatment	Trauma-Related Treatment
Systolic anterior motion	β blockade	Phenylephrine + volume
Hemorrhage	Transfusion of PRBC; fresh frozen plasma and platelets only as indicated	1:1.5:1 ratio of plasma/PRBC/platelet dose (massive) transfusion. rVIIa early
Hypotension	Volume, vasoactive agents to increase mean arterial blood pressure. Consider myocardial ischemia or exacerbation of preexisting disease (ie, CHF, valvular abnormalities)	No intervention if mean arterial blood pressure is >50 mm Hg (in absence of traumatic brain/spinal cord injury or known coronary artery disease) until hemorrhage control. Consider intraoperative TTE/TEE for traumatic cause (see **Table 1**)

SUMMARY

Patients with multiple severe injuries may present to the OR with little or no preoperative evaluation, and management strategies may differ from those for patients without trauma (**Table 3**). Hemorrhagic shock, gas exchange abnormalities, hemodynamic instability, and preexisting medical conditions are common. The use of damage control resuscitation, early factor replacement, and an understanding of the surgical priorities in trauma care can aid in the anesthetic management of this high-risk population.

ACKNOWLEDGMENTS

Mary Hyder, MD, Assistant Professor of Cardiac Trauma Anesthesiology, R Adams Cowley Shock Trauma Center, University of Maryland School of Medicine.

REFERENCES

1. Web-based injury statistics query and reporting system (WISQARS). US Department of Health and Human Services. CDC, National Center for Injury Prevention and Control, 2002.
2. Mathers CD, Loncar D. Updated projections of global mortality and burden of disease, 2002–2030: data sources, methods and results. Evidence and information for policy. Geneva: World Health Organization; 2005.
3. Fegheli NT, Prisant LM. Blunt myocardial injury. Chest 1995;108:1673–7.
4. Parmley LF, Mattingly TW, Manion WC, et al. Non penetrating traumatic injury of the aorta. Circulation 1958;17:1086–100.
5. Richens D, Kotidis K, Neale M, et al. Rupture of the aorta following road traffic accidents in the United Kingdom 1992–1999. The results of the co-operative crash injury study. Eur J Cardiothorac Surg 2003;23:143–8.
6. Synbrandy KC, Cramer MJM, Burgersdijk C. Diagnosing cardiac contusion: old wisdom and new insights. Heart 2003;89:485–9.
7. Bansal MK, Maraj S, Chewaproug D, et al. Myocardial contusion injury: redefining the diagnostic algorithm. Emerg Med J 2005;22:465–9.
8. McGillicuddy D, Rosen P. Diagnostic dilemmas and current controversies in blunt chest trauma. Emerg Med Clin North Am 2007;25:695–711.
9. Xenos ES, Abedi NN, Davenport DL, et al. Meta-analysis of endovascular vs open repair for traumatic descending thoracic aortic rupture. J Vasc Surg 2008;48(5):1343–51. Grade A.
10. Tang GL, Tehrani HY, Usman A, et al. Reduced mortality, paraplegia, and stroke with stent graft repair of blunt aortic transactions: a modern meta-analysis. J Vasc Surg 2008;47(3):671–5. Grade A.
11. Urgnani F, Lerut P, Da Rocha M, et al. Endovascular treatment of acute traumatic thoracic aortic injuries: a retrospective analysis of 20 cases. J Thorac Cardiovasc Surg 2009;138:1129–38.
12. Walsh SR, Tang TY, Sadat U, et al. Endovascular stenting versus open surgery for thoracic aortic disease: systemic review and meta-analysis of perioperative results. J Vasc Surg 2008;47(5):1094–8.
13. Vergez M, Pirracchio R, Mateo J, et al. Tako Tsubo cardiomyopathy in a patient with multiple trauma. Resuscitation 2009;80:1074–7.
14. Barleben A, Huerta S, Mendoza R, et al. Left ventricular injury with a normal pericardial window: case report and review of the literature. J Trauma 2007;63: 414–6.

15. Rootman DB, Latter D, Ahmed N. Case report of ventricular septal defect secondary to blunt chest trauma. Can J Surg 2007;50(3):227–8.
16. Rollins MD, Koehler RP, Stevens MH, et al. Traumatic ventricular septal defect: case report and review of the English literature since 1970. J Trauma 2005;58: 175–80.
17. Actis Dato GM, Arslanian A, Di Marzio P, et al. Posttraumatic and iatrogenic foreign bodies in the heart: report of fourteen cases and review of the literature. J Thorac Cardiovasc Surg 2003;126:408–14.
18. Bruschi G, Agati S, Iorio F, et al. Papillary muscle rupture and pericardial injuries after blunt chest trauma. Eur J Cardiothorac Surg 2001;20:200–2.
19. Simmers TA, Meijburg HWB, de la Riviere AB. Traumatic papillary muscle rupture. Ann Thorac Surg 2001;72:259–61.
20. Gunter L, Margreiter J, Jochberger S, et al. Systolic anterior motion of the mitral valve with left ventricular outflow tract obstruction: three cases of acute perioperative hypotension in noncardiac surgery. Anesth Analg 2005;100:1594–8.
21. Sherrid MV. Dynamic left ventricular outflow obstruction in hypertrophic cardiomyopathy revisited: significance, pathogenesis, and treatment. Cardiol Rev 1998;6:135–45.
22. Tayal VS, Beatty MA, Marx JA, et al. FAST (focused assessment with sonography in trauma) accurate for cardiac and intraperitoneal injury in penetrating anterior chest trauma. J Ultrasound Med 2004;23:457–72.
23. Salehia O, Teoh K, Mulji A. Blunt and penetrating cardiac trauma: a review. Can J Cardiol 2003;19:1054–9.
24. Fitzgerald M, Spencer J, Johnson F, et al. Definitive management of acute cardiac tamponade secondary to blunt trauma. Emerg Med Australas 2005; 17:494–9. Grade B.
25. Vignon P, Boncoeur M, Francois B, et al. Comparison of multiplane tranesophageal echocardiography and contrast-enhanced helical CT in the diagnosis of blunt traumatic cardiovascular injuries. Anesthesiology 2001;94:615–22.
26. Cinnella G, Dambrosio M, Brienza N, et al. Transesophageal echocardiography for diagnosis of traumatic aortic injury: an appraisal of the evidence. J Trauma 2004;57:1246–55.
27. Texeira PGR, Inaba K, Oncel D, et al. Blunt cardiac rupture: a 5-year NTDB analysis. J Trauma 2009;67:788–91.
28. Chaer RA, Doherty JC, Merlotti G, et al. A case of blunt injury to the superior vena cava and right atrial appendage: mechanisms of injury and review of the literature. Injury Extra 2005;36:341–5.
29. Demetriades D, Velhamos GC, Scalea TM, et al. Diagnosis and treatment of blunt thoracic aortic injuries: changing perspectives. J Trauma 2008;64:1415–8.
30. Smetana GW, Lawrence VA, Cornell JE, et al. Preoperative pulmonary risk stratification for noncardiothoracic surgery: systematic review for the American College of Physicians. Ann Intern Med 2006;144:581–95.
31. Lawrence VA, Cornell JE, Smetana GW, et al. Strategies to reduce postoperative pulmonary complications after noncardiothoracic surgery: systematic review for the American College of Physicians. Ann Intern Med 2006;144:596–608.
32. Manku K, Bacchetti P, Leung JM. Prognostic significance of postoperative in-hospital complications in elderly patients. I. Long-term survival. Anesth Analg 2003;96:583–9.
33. Miller PR, Croce MA, Bee TK, et al. ARDS after pulmonary contusion: accurate measurement of contusion volume identifies high-risk patients. J Trauma 2001; 51:223–8.

34. Cohn SM. Pulmonary contusion: review of the clinical entity. J Trauma 1997;42: 973–9.

35. Perl M, Gebhard F, Bruckner UB, et al. Pulmonary contusion causes impairment of macrophage and lymphocyte immune functions and increases mortality associated with a subsequent septic challenge. Crit Care Med 2005;33:1351–8.

36. McCunn M, Mauritz W, Sutcliffe A. Guidelines for management of mechanical ventilation in critically injured patients. Available at: http://www.itaccs.com/more/ventilation.htm. Accessed January 28, 2010.

37. Ullman DA, Fortune JB, Greenhouse BB, et al. The treatment of patients with multiple rib fractures using continuous thoracic epidural narcotic infusion. Reg Anesth 1989;14:43–7.

38. Bulger EM, Edwards T, Klotz P, et al. Epidural analgesia improves outcome after multiple rib fractures. Surgery 2004;136:426–30.

39. Peltier LF. Fat embolism. A current concept. Clin Orthop 1969;66:241–53.

40. Akhtar S. Fat embolism. Anesthesiol Clin 2009;27:533–50.

41. Djelouah I, Lefevre G, Ozier Y, et al. Fat embolism in orthopedic surgery: role of bone marrow fatty acid. Anesth Analg 1997;85:441–3.

42. Heine TA, Halambeck BL, Mark JB. Fatal pulmonary fat embolism in the early postoperative period. Anesthesiology 1998;89:1589–91.

43. Pape HC, Rixen D, Morley J, et al. EPOFF Study G. Impact of the method of initial stabilization for femoral shaft fractures in patients with multiple injuries at risk for complications (borderline patients). Ann Surg 2007;246:491–9.

44. ASA Practice Guidelines for Perioperative Blood Transfusion and Adjuvant Therapies. An updated report by the American Society of Anesthesiologists task force on perioperative blood transfusion and adjuvant therapies. Anesthesiology 2006;105:198–208.

45. Eisner MD, Thompson BT, Schoenfeld D, et al. Airway pressures and early barotrauma in patients with acute lung injury and acute respiratory distress syndrome. Am J Respir Crit Care Med 2002;165:978–82.

46. Boussarsar M, Thierry G, Jaber S, et al. Relationship between ventilatory settings and barotrauma in the acute respiratory distress syndrome. Intensive Care Med 2002;28:406–13.

47. Kauvar DS, Lefering R, Wade CE. Impact of hemorrhage on trauma outcome: an overview of epidemiology, clinical presentations, and therapeutic considerations. J Trauma 2006;60:S3–11.

48. Lefering R, Paffrath T, Linker R, et al. Head injury and outcome – what influence do concomitant injuries have? J Trauma 2008;65:1036–44.

49. Hortnagl H, Hammerle AF, Hackl JM, et al. The activity of the sympathetic nervous system following severe head injury. Intensive Care Med 1980;6:1–7.

50. Hamill RW, Woolf PD, McDonald JV, et al. Catecholamines predict outcome in trauma brain injury. Ann Neurol 1987;21:438–43.

51. Woolf PD, Hamill RW, Lee LA, et al. The predictive value of catecholamines in assessing outcome in trauma brain injury. J Neurosurg 1987;66:875–82.

52. Szerlip NJ, Bholat O, McCunn MM, et al. Extracorporeal life support as a treatment for neurogenic pulmonary edema and cardiac failure secondary to intractable intracranial hypertension: a case report and review of the literature [review]. J Trauma 2009;67:E69–71.

53. Yen TS, Liau CC, Chen YS, et al. Extracorporeal membrane oxygenation resuscitation for traumatic brain injury after decompressive craniotomy. Clin Neurol Neurosurg 2008;110:295–7.

54. Inaba K, Teixeira PG, David JS, et al. Beta-blockers in isolated blunt head injury. J Am Coll Surg 2008;206:432–8.

55. Arbabi S, Campion EM, Hemmila MR, et al. Beta-blocker use is associated with improved outcomes in adult trauma patients. J Trauma 2007;62:56–61.

56. Cotton BA, Snodgrass KB, Fleming SB, et al. Beta-blocker exposure is associated with improved survival after severe traumatic brain injury. J Trauma 2007; 62:26–33.

57. Zygun DA, Klortbeek JB, Fick GH, et al. Non-neurologic organ dysfunction in severe traumatic brain injury. Crit Care Med 2005;33:654–60.

58. Kemp CD, Johnson JC, Riordan WP, et al. How we die: the impact of nonneurologic organ dysfunction after severe traumatic brain injury. Am Surg 2008;74: 866–72.

59. Brain Trauma Foundation. Guidelines for the management of severe traumatic brain injury. J Neurotrauma 2007;24:S1–106.

60. Wing PC, Dalsey WC, Alvarez E, et al. Early acute management in adults with spinal cord injury. A clinical practice guideline for health-care professionals. J Spinal Cord Med 2008;31:408–79. Grade B.

61. Bickell WH, Wall MJ Jr, Pepe PE, et al. Immediate versus delayed fluid resuscitation for hypotensive patients with penetrating torso injuries. N Engl J Med 1994;331:1105–9. Grade A.

62. Dutton RP, Mackenzie CF, Scalea TM. Hypotensive resuscitation during active hemorrhage: impact on in-hospital mortality. J Trauma 2002;52:1141–6. Grade A.

63. Yaghoubian A, Lewis RJ, Putnam B, et al. Reanalysis of prehospital intravenous fluid administration in patients with penetrating truncal injury and field hypotension. Am Surg 2007;73:1027–30. Grade B.

64. Stern SA. Low-volume fluid resuscitation for presumed hemorrhagic shock: helpful or harmful? Curr Opin Crit Care 2001;7:422–30.

65. Spinella PC, Holcomb JB. Resuscitation and transfusion principles for traumatic hemorrhage. Blood Rev 2009;23:231–40.

66. Brohi K, Singh J, Heron M. Acute traumatic coagulopathy. J Trauma 2003;54: 1127–30.

67. MacLeod JB, Lynn M, McKenney MG, et al. Early coagulopathy predicts mortality in trauma. J Trauma 2003;55:39–44.

68. Brohi K, Cohen MJ, Ganter MT, et al. Acute traumatic coagulopathy: initiated by hypoperfusion: modulated through the protein C pathway? Ann Surg 2007;245:812–8.

69. Hess JR, Brohi K, Dutton RP, et al. The coagulopathy of trauma: a review of mechanisms. J Trauma 2008;65:748–54.

70. Como JJ, Dutton RP, Scalea TM, et al. Blood transfusion rates in the care of acute trauma. Transfusion 2004;44:809–13.

71. Dutton RP, Lefering R, Lynn M. Database predictors of transfusion and mortality. J Trauma 2006;60:S70–7.

72. Holcomb JB, Wade CE, Michalek JE, et al. Increased plasma and platelet to red blood cell ratios improves outcome in 466 massively transfused civilian trauma patients. Ann Surg 2008;248:447–58.

73. Stinger HK, Spinella PC, Perkins JG, et al. The ratio of fibrinogen to red cells transfused affects survival in casualties receiving massive transfusions at an Army combat support hospital. J Trauma 2008;64:S79–85.

74. Borgman MA, Spinella PC, Perkins JG, et al. The ratio of blood products transfused affects mortality in patients receiving massive transfusions at a combat surgical support hospital. J Trauma 2007;63:805–13.

75. Duchesne JC, Islam TM, Stuke L, et al. Hemostatic resuscitation during surgery improves survival in patients with traumatic-induced coagulopathy. J Trauma 2009;67:33–9.
76. Sperry JL, Ochoa JB, Gunn SR, et al. An FFP: PRBC transfusion ratio >1:1.5 is associated with a lower risk of mortality after massive transfusion. J Trauma 2008;65:986–93.
77. Scalea TM, Bochiccho KM, Lumpkins K, et al. Early aggressive use of fresh frozen plasma does not improve outcome in critically injured trauma patients. Ann Surg 2008;248:578–84.
78. Watson GA, Sperry JL, Rosengart MR, et al. Fresh frozen plasma is independently associated with a higher risk of multiple organ failure and acute respiratory distress syndrome. J Trauma 2009;67:221–30.
79. Malone DL, Dunne J, Tracy JK, et al. Blood transfusion, independent of shock severity, is associated with worse outcome in trauma. J Trauma 2003;54: 898–905 [discussion: 905–7].
80. Vincent JL, Baron JF, Reinhart K, et al. Anemia and blood transfusion in critically ill patients. JAMA 2002;288:1499–507.
81. Taylor RW, Manganaro L, O'Brien J, et al. Impact of allogenic packed red blood cell transfusion on nosocomial infection rates in the critically ill patient. Crit Care Med 2002;30:2249–54.
82. Dunne JR, Riddle MS, Danko J, et al. Blood transfusion is associated with infection and increased resource utilization in combat casualties. Am Surg 2006;72:619.
83. Alam HB, Rhee P. New developments in fluid resuscitation. Surg Clin North Am 2007;87:55–72.
84. Cotton BA, Guy JS, Morris JA Jr, et al. The cellular, metabolic, and systemic consequences of aggressive fluid resuscitation strategies. Shock 2006;26:115–21.
85. Deb S, Sun L, Martin B, et al. Lactated Ringer's solution and hetastarch but not plasma resuscitation after rat hemorrhagic shock is associated with immediate lung apoptosis by the up-regulation of the Bax protein. J Trauma 2000;49:47–55.
86. Kiraly LN, Differding JA, Enomoto TM, et al. Resuscitation with normal saline (NS) vs. lactated ringers (LR) modulates hypercoagulability and leads to increased blood loss in an uncontrolled hemorrhagic shock swine model. J Trauma 2006;61:57–64.
87. Balogh Z, McKinley BA, Cocanour CS, et al. Supranormal trauma resuscitation causes more cases of abdominal compartment syndrome. Arch Surg 2003;138: 637–43.
88. Wiedemann HP, Wheeler AP, Bernard GR, et al. National Heart, Lung, and Blood Institute Acute Respiratory Distress Syndrome (ARDS) Clinical Trials Network. Comparison of two fluid-management strategies in acute lung injury. N Engl J Med 2006;354:2564–75.
89. Boucher BA, Traub O. Achieving hemostasis in the surgical field. Pharmacotherapy 2009;29:2S–7S.
90. Kessler CM, Ortel TL. Recent developments in topical thrombins. Thromb Haemost 2009;102:15–24.
91. Schreiber MA, Tieu B. Hemostasis in operation Iraqi freedom III. Surgery 2007; 142:S61–6.
92. Sohn VY, Eckert MJ, Arthrus ZM, et al. Efficacy of three topical hemostatic agents applied by medics in a lethal groin injury model. J Surg Res 2009;154:258–61.
93. Duchesne JC, Mathew KA, Marr AB, et al. Current evidence based guidelines for factor VIIa use in trauma: the good, the bad and the ugly. Am Surg 2008; 74:1159–65.

94. Dutton RP, McCunn M, Hyder M, et al. Factor VIIa for control of hemorrhage: early experience in critically ill trauma patients. J Trauma 2004;57:709–19.
95. Boffard KD, Riou B, Warren B, et al. Recombinant factor VIIA as adjunctive therapy for bleeding control in severely injured trauma patients: two parallel randomized, placebo-controlled, double-blind clinical trials. J Trauma 2005; 59:8–15.
96. Perkins JG, Schreiber MA, Wade CE. Early versus late recombinant factor VIIa in combat trauma patients requiring massive transfusion. J Trauma 2007;62: 1095–101.
97. Stein DM, Dutton RP, Hess JR, et al. Low-dose rVIIa for trauma patients with coagulapathy. Injury 2008;39:1054–61.
98. Stein DM, Dutton RP, Kramer ME, et al. Reversal of coagulopathy in critically ill patients with trauma brain injury: rVIIa is more cost-effective than plasma. J Trauma 2009;66:63–75.
99. Stein DM, Dutton RP, Kramer ME, et al. Recombinant factor VIIa: decreasing time to intervention in coagulopathic patients with severe traumatic brain injury. J Trauma 2008;64:620–8.
100. Pape HC, Giannoudis PV, Krettek C, et al. Timing of fixation of major fractures in blunt polytrauma: role of conventional indicators in clinical decision making. J Orthop Trauma 2005;19:551–62.
101. Tuttle MS, Smith WR, Williams AE, et al. Safety and efficacy of damage control external fixation versus early definitive stabilization for femoral shaft fractures in the multiple-injured patient. J Trauma 2009;67:602–5.
102. Scalea TM, Boswell SA, Scott JD, et al. External fixation as a bridge to intramedullary mailing for patients with multiple injuries and with femur fractures: damage control orthopedics. J Trauma 2000;48:613–21.
103. Pape HC, Tornetta P, Tarkin I, et al. Timing of fracture fixation in multitrauma patients: the role of early total care and damage control surgery. J Am Acad Orthop Surg 2009;17:541–9.
104. Giannoudis PV, Abbott C, Stone M, et al. Fatal systemic inflammatory response syndrome following early bilateral femoral nailing. Intensive Care Med 1998;24: 641–2.
105. Cothren CC, Osborn PM, Moore EE, et al. Preperitoneal pelvic packing for hemodynamically unstable pelvic fractures: a paradigm shift. J Trauma 2007; 62:834–9.
106. Olson SA, Burgess A. Classification and initial management of patients with unstable pelvic ring injuries. Instr Course Lect 2005;54:383–93.
107. Anderson HL 3rd, Shapiro MB, Delius RE, et al. Extracorporeal life support for respiratory failure after multiple trauma. J Trauma 1994;37:266–72.
108. Barreda E, Flecher E, Aubert S, et al. Extracorporeal life support in right ventricular rupture secondary to blast injury. Interact Cardiovasc Thorac Surg 2007;6:87–8.
109. Seiji M, Sadaki I, Shigeaki I, et al. The efficacy of rewarming with a portable and percutaneous cardiopulmonary bypass system in accidental deep hypothermia patients with hemodynamic instability. J Trauma 2008;65:1391–5.
110. Maggio P, Hemmila M, Haft J, et al. Extracorporeal life support for massive pulmonary embolism. J Trauma 2007;62:570–6.
111. McCunn M, Reynolds HN, Cottingham CA, et al. Extracorporeal support in an adult with severe carbon monoxide poisoning and shock following smoke inhalation: a case report. Perfusion 2000;15:169–73.
112. Michaels AJ, Schriener RJ, Kolla S, et al. Extracorporeal life support in pulmonary failure after trauma. J Trauma 1999;46:638–45.

113. Perchinsky MJ, Long WB, Hill JG, et al. Extracorporeal cardiopulmonary life support with heparin-bonded circuitry in the resuscitation of massively injured trauma patients. Am J Surg 1995;169:488–91.
114. Huang YK, Liu KS, Lu MS, et al. Extracorporeal life support in post-traumatic respiratory distress patients. Resuscitation 2009;80:535–9.
115. Madershahian N, Wittwer T, Strauch J, et al. Application of ECMO in multi-trauma patients with ARDS as rescue therapy. J Cardiovasc Surg 2007;22: 180–4.
116. Flörchinger B, Philipp A, Klose A, et al. Pumpless extracorporeal lung assist: a 10-year institutional experience. Ann Thorac Surg 2008;86:410–7.
117. Kuhne CA, Ruchholtz S, Kaiser GM, et al. Mortality in severely injured elderly trauma patients – when does age become a risk factor? World J Surg 2005; 29:1476–82.
118. Wutzler S, Maegele M, Marzi I, et al. Association of preexisting medical conditions with in-hospital mortality in multiple-trauma patients. J Am Coll Surg 2009; 209:75–81.
119. Wutzler S, Lefering R, Laurer HL, et al. Changes in geriatric traumatology: an analysis of 14,869 patients from the German trauma registry. Unfallchirurg 2008;111:592–8.
120. Bercault N, Boulain T, Kuteifan K, et al. Obesity-related excess mortality rate in an adult intensive care unit: a risk-adjusted matched cohort study. Crit Care Med 2004;32:998–1003.
121. Neville AL, Brown CV, Weng J, et al. Obesity is an independent risk factor of mortality in severely injured blunt trauma patients. Arch Surg 2004;139:983–7.
122. Byrnes MC, McDaniel MD, Moore MB, et al. The effect of obesity on outcomes among injured patients. J Trauma 2005;58:232–7.
123. Chen ZB, Ni LM, Gao Y, et al. Pre-existing cirrhosis is associated with increased mortality of traumatic patients: analysis of cases from a trauma center in east China. World J Gastroenterol 2007;13:5654–8.
124. Christmas AB, Wilson AK, Franklin GA, et al. Cirrhosis and trauma: a deadly duo. Am Surg 2005;71:996–1000.
125. Dangleben DA, Jazaeri O, Wasser T, et al. Impact of cirrhosis on outcomes in trauma. J Am Coll Surg 2006;203:908–13.
126. Frink M, Pape HC, van Griensven M, et al. Influence of sex and age on mods and cytokines after multiple injuries. Shock 2007;27:151–6.

Patients Presenting with Acute Toxin Ingestion

Gary E. Hill, MD, FCCM*, Babatunde Ogunnaike, MD, Dawood Nasir, MD

KEYWORDS

- Toxins • Anesthesia • Toxicity • Drug Effects
- Poisonings • Envenomations

Organ toxicity caused by poisons or drug therapy is diverse and, in many cases, not commonly encountered clinically. In general, commonly encountered conditions caused by drug/toxin pharmacology can be categorized by shared mechanisms of organ injury. The following discussion of drug/toxin-induced injury is divided into 7 categories based on shared pathophysiology of the offending toxin or therapeutic drug administration and the likelihood of being encountered by the clinician: (1) QT interval prolongation and drug-induced channelopathies; (2) acquired methemoglobinemia; (3) drugs causing hyperthermic syndromes, alcohol (ethanol)-induced injuries and herbal drug abuse injuries; (4) drug toxicity in the chronic pain patient and dextromethorphan (DMP) toxicity; (5) poisonings causing metabolic acidosis, including carbon monoxide; (6) military/terrorist poisonings, including botulism and Botox; and (7) poisonous bites and envenomations.

QT INTERVAL PROLONGATION AND DRUG-INDUCED CHANNELOPATHIES

A 34-year-old man scheduled for elective surgery is currently treated with methadone for heroine addiction. He presents the day of surgery with a serum potassium level of 3.0 mEq/L and an electrocardiograph (ECG) shows a QTc interval (corrected by the Bazett formula: QTc = QT/$\sqrt{RR}$) of 500 milliseconds with a prominent U wave. *What would you do next?*

The cardiac action potential (AP) is generated by ion flows across cell membranes through specific ion channels. Phase 0 depolarization is developed by an inward sodium current and this inward current is responsible for striking the R wave on the surface ECG (**Fig. 1**). Thus, a drug that primarily blocks the sodium channel (lidocaine) can slur or prolong the QRS complex. The T wave is struck by ventricular

Department of Anesthesiology and Pain Management, the University of Texas Southwestern Medical Center, 5323 Harry Hines Boulevard, Dallas, TX 75390-9068, USA
* Corresponding author.
E-mail address: gary.hill@utsouthwestern.edu

Anesthesiology Clin 28 (2010) 117–137
doi:10.1016/j.anclin.2010.01.002
1932-2275/10/$ – see front matter © 2010 Elsevier Inc. All rights reserved.

anesthesiology.theclinics.com

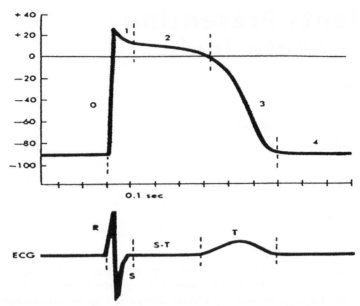

Fig. 1. The relationship of the phases of the cardiac AP with the surface ECG. Phase 0 (inward sodium current) strikes the R wave, phase 3 repolarization strikes the T wave. Sodium channel blockade will slur and prolong the QRS complex; potassium channel blockade will prolong phase 3 repolarization and lengthen the QT interval.

repolarization, which is caused by an outward potassium current (phase 3 repolarization). As **Fig. 1** shows, a major determinant of the total action potential duration (APD) (onset of phase 0 to the end of phase 3) is the duration of phase 3 repolarization.[1] The APD is determined clinically by measuring the QT interval, which, in turn, is a measure of conduction velocity. When conduction velocity slows (QT interval is prolonged) as a result of a drug effect or electrolyte effects, this can present a physiologic condition promoting the appearance of arrhythmias.

The primary potassium channels that are responsible for phase 3 repolarization are the rapid potassium current channel and the delayed rectifier current channel; the latter channel is encoded by the human ether-a-go-go (HERG) gene and is almost exclusively the channel that all of the drugs currently discussed bind to and inhibit, thereby prolonging the QTc interval. Immediately following phase 3 repolarization and before the onset of a new AP, small spontaneous inward calcium currents normally occur and are called early after depolarizations (EADs). If the conduction velocity is slowed (prolonged QTc), these EADs can summate into a positive depolarization wave at the end of phase 3, creating a U wave on the surface ECG. If the U wave achieves enough depolarization to reach threshold levels, a new R wave will be generated, creating an R on T event, thus potentially triggering a reentrant ventricular arrhythmia. This mechanism is believed to be responsible for developing the unique polymorphic ventricular tachycardia referred to as torsades de pointes (TdP).[2]

TdP was first described in 1964 in patients receiving the class 1A antiarrhythmic drug quinidine. A continually growing list of drugs are reported to inhibit the HERG potassium channel and cause QTc prolongation and potentially create a TdP type of arrhythmia (**Table 1**). The drugs specifically of interest to the anesthesiologist include cocaine, droperidol, sevoflurane, haloperidol, ondansetron, methadone, and all local anesthetics (with the exception of lidocaine, which does not block potassium

| Table 1 |
| Drugs known to prolong QT interval and potentially cause TdP |
Category	Drug
Antiarrhythmics	Vaughn-Williams class 1A Disopyramide, procainamide, quinidine 1C Encainide, flecainide III Amiodarone (TdP rare), dofetilide, ibutilide, sotalol
Calcium channel–blocking drugs	Diltiazem, verapamil
Psychiatric	Amitriptyline, chlorpromaxine, desipramine, fluxetine, haloperidol, imipramine, lithium, pimozide, paraxetine, sertraline, thioridazine, ziprasidone
Antihistamines	Astemizole, diphenhydramine, hydroxyzine, terfenadine
Antiinfective	Amantadine, ciprofloxacin, chloroquine, clarithromycin, erythromycin, fluconazole, grepafloxacin, itraconazole, ketoconazole, pentamidine, quinine
Antiretroviral	Amprenavir, indinavir, ritonavir
Anesthetic Drugs	Inhaled agents (sevo- and desflurane), methadone, droperidol, ondansetron, cocaine, all LAs (except lidocaine), hypokalemia especially acute onset (hyperventilation, infusions of bicarbonate, insulin, epinephrine), vasopressin, organophosphates

channels). Potassium channel blockade (prolongation of phase 3 depolarization and therefore APD) is necessary to significantly prolong the QTc interval and potentially cause TdP.[3] Extracellular hypokalemia will also prolong the QTc interval by hyperpolarizing the resting membrane potential, therefore requiring a longer phase 3 repolarization period, and thus prolonging APD and QTc (**Fig. 2**).[1] Hypokalemia will potentiate drug-induced QTc prolongation and enhance the incidence of TdP.[4] In addition, an estimated 1 in 10,000 individuals is a carrier of the long QT syndrome gene (congenital LQTS) and routine ECG screening may show a normal QT interval in these individuals. Congenital LQTS may be unmasked by synergism on the introduction of a drug that blocks potassium channels; for example, the onset of TdP and sudden death in

$$E = 60 \cdot \log \frac{[K]_o}{[K]_i}.$$

or

$$E = -61 \cdot \log \frac{K_I}{K_o}$$

Fig. 2. The Nernst equation shows that the ratio of extracellular potassium (K_o) to intracellular potassium (K_i) is the primary determinant of the resting membrane potential (E). Chronic reduction of K_o by thiazide diuretics or acute reduction of K_o with simultaneous increase of K_i (hyperventilation, infusion of insulin, epinephrine, or bicarbonate) will hyperpolarize (make more negative) the E and require a longer phase 3 repolarization to return to baseline resting membrane potential. This process will prolong AP duration and, by definition, lengthen the QT interval.

a recreational (first-time) user of cocaine. Prolongation of the QT interval is now the most common cause of withdrawal of a drug from the market following approval by the US Food and Drug Administration (FDA). Drugs associated with QT prolongation include antipsychotics (lithium, haloperidol, and chlorpromazine), antihistamines (diphenhydramine and astemizole), and antiinfective drugs (erythromycin, clarithromycin, chloroquine). The effects of these drugs on the HERG channel are synergistic, and, along with electrolyte disturbance (hypokalemia/magnesemia), may summate into a fatal TdP type of arrhythmia. Although no absolutes are defined, a QTc interval approaching or greater than 500 milliseconds is an absolute red flag warning that TdP is an increasingly likely event.[3]

Cocaine

Because a large percentage of Americans 12 years of age or older (14% of the total population of the United States) have tried cocaine at least once, it is likely that the clinician will be required to give medical care to a cocaine-positive patient. Cocaine can cause coronary spasm, accelerated atherosclerosis, increased plasma catecholamines (by reuptake inhibition of norepinephrine), myocardial ischemia, and aortic dissection, so the report that 43% of cocaine users experience arrhythmia within 12 hours of cocaine ingestion[5] is not surprising. Although more than 80% of cocaine abusers have an abnormal ECG, ECG findings specific for ischemia or infarction are infrequent (2%–6%). Increasingly frequent reports of QTc prolongation and TdP are explained by the known sodium and potassium (HERG) channel–blocking effects of cocaine. The importance of this cocaine-induced channelopathy is demonstrated by the shortening (improvement) of the QTc interval by the administration of sodium ion (sodium bicarbonate),[6] thus antagonizing the cocaine-induced sodium channel blockade. A similar pharmacologic comparison would be giving calcium ion to a patient with an overdose of a calcium channel–blocking drug. The sodium and potassium channel blockade caused by cocaine resembles that caused by the Vaughn-Williams antiarrhythmic class 1c drug flecainide, the use of which has largely been abandoned because of TdP generation.[7] Cocaine may unmask unrecognized and undiagnosed congenital LQTS by causing TdP and arrhythmia generation in this group of patients, explaining some of the reports of sudden death during the first-time recreational use of cocaine.

Clinical management of the cocaine-positive patient, in addition to the well-known avoidance of β-blocking drugs (including labetalol), and avoidance of drugs known to prolong APD and thus QTc (see later discussion), would be prudent. Because propofol, midazolam, synthetic opioids (fentanyl, sufentanil), neuromuscular blocking drugs, and nitrous oxide are reported to have no effect on APD, the clinician is allowed a reasonable choice of agents and a regional technique with lidocaine.

Methadone

Methadone is now the most common drug associated with TdP at Parkland Hospital in Dallas, Texas. A recent study found more than 16% of patients receiving methadone had significant QTc prolongation compared with 0% in controls, with nearly 4% of patients receiving methadone experiencing TdP. This study also showed that hypokalemia is a significant synergistic risk factor for TdP generation.[8]

Local Anesthetics (Except Lidocaine)

Bupivacaine, ropivacaine, and mepivacaine bind to and inhibit potassium channels and therefore prolong APD and the surface ECG QTc interval duration.[9] Reports of synergism of potassium channel blockade properties between mutant potassium channels (congenital LQTS) and local anesthetics (LAs) suggest that regional anesthesia with the LAs mentioned earlier should be approached with caution in all patients with QTc approaching 450 to 500 milliseconds. The LAs listed earlier should be used with caution in patients known to be receiving any drug known to prolong the QTc. If a regional technique with one of these LAs is pursued, continual ECG monitoring following LA injection, and continuing until the regional block is dissipated, would enhance patient safety.

Sevo- and Desflurane

These inhaled agents are known to block potassium channels and therefore prolong cardiac APD and QTc.[10] Sevoflurane has been shown to synergize with the class 3 antiarrhythmic drugs sotalol and dofetilide in APD prolongation, demonstrating the necessity of the clinician to be aware of the current medication history and the effects of those drugs on QTc for those patients receiving inhaled agents.

Antiemetics

Droperidol causes a dose-dependent prolongation of the APD and QTc by blocking the HERG potassium channel.[11] Ondansetron is reported to have similar effects. Although arrhythmia generation is highly unlikely following small (1.25 mg or less) antiemetic doses, the usual caveat must be remembered: all drugs that block HERG channels are synergistic. Therefore, in patients currently ingesting drugs known to prolong QTc, even with a preoperative ECG showing the QTc to be less than 500 milliseconds, it may be prudent for the clinician to avoid droperidol and ondansetron and use other antiemetic drugs known to be without QTc effects (eg, dexamethasone) in those patients with a QTc greater than 450 milliseconds.

In conclusion, surgery in the case described at the start of this section should be cancelled, his hypokalemia corrected, and the dose of methadone reevaluated. A QTc approaching or greater than 500 milliseconds is a red flag for TdP and should not be ignored. If surgery is urgent, any drug already discussed that prolongs QTc should be avoided, as should hyperventilation (which causes a rapid extracellular hypokalemia, see **Fig. 2**); serum potassium levels should be increased with supplemental intravenous (IV) potassium. If a regional technique is chosen, lidocaine would be the LA of choice.

ACQUIRED METHEMOGLOBINEMIA

A 66-year-old man presented for emergency exploratory laparotomy for free intraabdominal air. Medication history included oral isosorbide dinitrate for ischemic heart disease. His wife also confirmed the use of Lanacane (20% benzocaine) topical spray (purchased over the counter) for recent sunburn pain and intraorally for painful mucosal ulcers caused by poorly fitting dentures. In the emergency room it was noted that his pulse oximeter read 85% to 86% despite high inhaled oxygen concentrations. Arterial blood gas (ABG) revealed an arterial Po_2 of 94%. *What would you do next?*

Methemoglobin (MHgb) is the oxidized (Fe^{3+}) form of iron in the hemoglobin molecule, and in this state cannot bind and transport oxygen. In addition, the oxyhemoglobin dissociation curve is left-shifted, thus reducing the peripheral unloading of O_2.[12] The action of cytochrome b5 methemoglobin reductase normally keeps MHgb levels less than 2%. Cytochrome b5 methemoglobin reductase is also dependent on reduced nicotine adenine dinucleotide phosphate diaphorase (methylene blue enhances the activity of this enzyme and it is generally understood that this enzyme reduces methylene blue to leukomethylene blue; leukomethylene blue then reduces MHgb to Hgb).[13]

The most common class of drugs used clinically that cause MHgb are the LAs, which are considered indirect oxidizers; that is, in vivo metabolism of LAs produce amine metabolites that are the actual oxidizers.[14] The LAs known to cause MHgb are lidocaine (rare and unlikely), mepivacaine (also unlikely), tetracaine, prilocaine (likely), and benzocaine (highly likely). Intraoral spraying of benzocaine during the inhalation phase shows rapid transmucosal airway absorption and has resulted in measured MHgb levels as high as 60%.[15]

Methemoglobinemia is diagnosed by MHgb levels greater than 2% or the Kronenberg test, which is a simple visual evaluation performed by dropping side by side normal blood (to serve as a visual contrast or control) and MHgb blood. The failure of the MHgb blood to change from the typical chocolate brown color following room air exposure or exposure to O_2 to a color matching that of the normal control blood drop would constitute a positive test for MHgb.[16] Skin color, although certainly not diagnostic, has been described as black, gray, chocolate/brownish, purple, or pale. Blood color has been described as chocolate/brown, black, burgundy, red, cyanotic, or blue/purple. Oxygen saturation measured by standard dual (2 wave length) pulse oximetry has been reported to vary between 50% and 94%, with a median of 85%. An important finding and clue to correct diagnosis is the finding of a disconnection (of the expected Spo_2/arterial Po_2 relationship) between a simultaneously measured pulse oximetric oxygen saturation of less than 90% while the directly measured (by standard Clark electrode) arterial Pao_2 is greater than 70 mm Hg. A normal (standard) oxyhemoglobin dissociation curve would couple an Spo_2 of 90% with an arterial Po_2 of 60 mm Hg.

A common finding is the concomitant use of another oxidizing drug such as nitrate therapy, trimethoprim-sulfamethoxazole (bactrim), dapsone, phenazopyridine, and phenacetin.[14] Reported complications of MHgb include myocardial infarction (in particular non-Q wave infarction with cardiac enzyme elevation), coma, seizures, respiratory failure, shock, and hypoxic cerebral injury. Most patients with MHgb greater than 8% are symptomatic. Standard (dual wave length) pulse oximeters may grossly underestimate the degree of systemic hypoxemia, whereas CO-oximeters with multiple (usually 8) light wavelengths would give a more accurate estimation of the true Spo_2 and the %MHgb.[17]

Prilocaine is metabolized to *ortho*-toluidine, which is responsible for Hgb oxidation to MHgb. Infants less than 6 months old are more susceptible to oxidation because of lower enzymatic levels of NADH, thus prilocaine should be avoided in this age group. Because no difference in doses of benzocaine exists between a therapeutic dose and a toxic dose and because of the difficulty in predicting which patient will develop significant MHgb with exposure, it has been suggested that the clinical use of benzocaine should be restricted or abandoned.[18] In 2006 the Veterans Affairs Central Pharmacy recommended that lidocaine be used for topical anesthesia for airway procedures and that benzocaine-containing topical sprays should not be used and should be removed from hospital pharmacy inventories.

The case described at the start of this section had a measured MHgb of 18% and was successfully treated with methylene blue (1 mg/kg)[19] with a prompt (within 60 minutes) improvement of the pulse oximeter (standard 2 wave length) reading to 96% to 97%. The remainder of the hospital course was uneventful following a diverting colostomy for a perforated colonic diverticulum.

DRUGS CAUSING HYPERTHERMIC SYNDROMES, ALCOHOL (ETHANOL)-INDUCED INJURIES, AND HERBAL DRUG ABUSE INJURIES

A 25-year-old woman presents to your critical care service after collapsing at a night-club. Her past medical history includes Zoloft (setraline) and over-the-counter St John's wort for depression. She admits to ingesting Ecstasy [3,4-methylenedioxyme-thamphetamine (MDMA)] and "a couple of lines" of cocaine. She is combative, disoriented, uncooperative, has leg and arm rigidity, and her vital signs include blood pressure (BP) of 185/105, heart rate (HR) 135, and temperature 39.9°C. ECG shows sinus tachycardia with normal QTc interval and isoelectric ST segments. *What would you do next?*

Toxin-induced hyperthermic syndromes must be included in the differential diagnosis of any patient presenting with muscle rigidity and fever. It is important for the clinician to recognize the underlying cause of drug (toxin)-induced hyperthermic syndromes because proper treatment will vary depending on the cause.

Norepinephrine, dopamine, and serotonin are all neurotransmitters that effect hypothalamic control of body temperature. Drugs or toxins that alter brain concentrations of these neurotransmitters are capable of altering body temperature regulation. Cocaine, amphetamine, methamphetamine, and MDMA are known to cause the serotonin syndrome (SS), especially when combined with antidepressants.[20] With the common use of selective serotonin reuptake inhibitors (SSRIs) prescribed for clinical depression and the increased recreational use of the illegal drugs listed earlier (especially MDMA), a dramatic increase in the SS is being reported. The earliest case report of the SS (1955) was attributed to the combination of meperidine (Demerol) and the monoamine oxidase inhibitor (MAOI) iproniazid. The most widely reported case of the SS occurred in 1984 when 18-year-old Libby Zion died of an SS caused by the combination of meperidine and phenelzine (an MAOI).[21] This death resulted in regulations requiring restriction of resident physician working hours, increased faculty supervision of residents, and controls for the use of patient restraints.

Most patients with the SS present with a combination of altered mental status (coma, confusion, agitation, seizures), abnormal neuromuscular activity (rigidity, myoclonus), and autonomic instability (fever, diaphoresis, tachycardia, hypertension). If the SS includes rhabdomyolysis, metabolic acidosis, coagulopathy, and marked temperature elevation (>43°C), the mortality rate is significantly increased. Many drugs, including MAOIs, amphetamines, MDMA, cocaine, tricyclic antidepressants, SSRIs, tramadol, meperidine, lithium, L-dopa, and lysergic acid diethylamide (LSD), among others, increase brain serotonin levels and thus may cause the SS.[22] Increased ambient temperature (incidence of the SS peak in the summer) and motor activity (all-night dance parties) will enhance the development of the SS syndrome following the use of any drug known to increase brain serotonin levels. In addition, a significant increase in the plasma levels of catecholamines (primarily norepinephrine, with the accompanying cardiovascular effects) are reported following MDMA, amphetamine, and cocaine ingestion.[23]

Therapy for the SS (as the case report at the start of this section was managed) would include external cooling, a combined α- and β-blocking drug (carvedilol) or calcium channel–blocking drugs for the sympathetic instability (hypertension and tachycardia), and benzodiazepines (midazolam) and propofol (by infusion) for control of the central nervous system (CNS) symptoms.[24]

The neuroleptic malignant syndrome (NMS) may be difficult to distinguish clinically from the SS. The NMS is normally seen following use of high-potency neuroleptics, such as haloperidol, but has been reported with the use of metaclopramide (Reglan),[25] promethazine, or following the withdrawal of antiparkinson drug therapy. Dantrolene (alone or combined with bromocriptine) is a commonly recommended therapy for NMS.

Malignant hyperthermia (MH), a well-known syndrome in the anesthesia community, is also characterized by sympathetic instability with significant elevations in plasma catecholamines. Increased survival in MH animal models has been reported following the use of α-blocking drugs.

Alcohol (Ethanol)-Induced Injuries

Alcohol abuse causes multiple injuries including stroke, cardiomyopathy, arrhythmias, intracerebral and subarachnoid hemorrhage (secondary to hypertension), accelerated atherosclerosis, aortic dissection, myocardial infarction, and hypertension, whereas light alcohol use is reported to reduce these complications. Currently alcohol abuse is considered the leading cause of nonischemic cardiomyopathy (referred to as alcoholic heart muscle disease)[26]; 11% of total hospitalizations for heart failure are considered secondary to alcohol consumption. Up to 30% of new onset atrial fibrillation have been found to be caused by alcohol consumption.[27]

Herbal Drug Injuries

It is estimated that 42% of the population uses alternative treatments and over-the-counter supplements. In 1994, legislation was passed that classified dietary supplements as foods, exempting them from safety standards to which prescription and over-the-counter drugs must adhere, thus increasing their availability to the general population. Although numerous herbal products are widely available, this discussion is limited to ephedra and St John's wort.

Ephedra

The availability of ephedra continues despite FDA alerts and rulings prohibiting the sale of dietary supplements containing ephedra. Although ephedra has been used for at least 5000 years in Chinese medicine, it is primarily used in the United States for weight loss or to increase energy levels. Although ephedrine was isolated from ephedra in 1887, ephedra also is known to contain pseudoephedrine, methylephedrine, norephedrine, methylpseudoephedrine, and norpseudoephedrine (all sympathomimetic alkaloids).[28] Ephedra is commonly combined with caffeine, forming a product that has significant agonism at the α and β adrenergic receptors and indirect agonism by augmenting norepinephrine release. Because of a large variation in the concentrations of ephedrine alkaloids present in supplements, significant cardiovascular response variation will be observed following ingestion. A common street name for ephedra in Dallas, TX, is herbal ecstasy. The euphoric and stimulant effects of ephedra are less intense but similar to the amphetamines. Anxiety, arrhythmia, palpitations, headaches, intracranial hemorrhage, hypertension, seizures, stroke, myocardial infarction, hyperthermia, and death have all been reported following ephedra use.[29] In fact, myocardial infarction secondary to isolated coronary artery vasospasm has been documented following ephedra ingestion in patients with normal coronary arteries.

St John's Wort

The concentration of the active constituents of St John's wort, hypericin and hyperforin, vary greatly from plant to plant, but commercial preparations are standardized to between 0.2% and 0.5% for the former constituent and 3%

for the latter. Because hypericin is known to be an MAOI, inhibiting catechol-*O*-methyltransferase and the reuptake of serotonin, dopamine, and norepinephrine (thus raising brain monoamine levels), this explains its popularity as a treatment of depression and anxiety.[30]

St John's wort is an inducer of the cytochrome P450 liver enzyme systems, altering the metabolism of many drugs coadministered with the wort. There is an increased clearance of midazolam and alprazolam. Studies show a low incidence of side effects, including no effect on the QTc interval.

The problem with St John's wort is the frequent reports of interactions between herbs and prescription drugs. The SS has been reported with the concomitant use of other serotonergic drugs, as in the case described at the start of this section. In addition, decreased plasma levels of digoxin, verapamil, warfarin, methadone, cyclosporine, theophylline, amitriptyline, midazolam, alprazolam, omeprazole, and simvastatin have been reported with concomitant *Hypericum* use. Reactions from delayed emergence to cardiovascular collapse during and following general anesthesia (accomplished with fentanyl, propofol, and sevoflurance) have been reported in patients using St John's wort.

DRUG TOXICITY IN THE CHRONIC PAIN PATIENT AND DMP TOXICITY

A 60-year-old man presents to your chronic pain management clinic for control of low-back pain that was not successfully treated with 3 lumbar laminectomies, the last including bone fusion and hardware placement. He has a past history including IV drug and alcohol abuse and is hepatitis C positive. He admits to taking 6 to 9 tablets of Lorcet (**Table 2**) routinely during a 24-hour period. His current complaints include postprandial epigastric pain, right upper quadrant tenderness, anorexia, nausea, occasional vomiting, and weight loss. Laboratory studies report an aspartate aminotransferase (AST) plasma concentration of 324 IU/L (normal range 10–50 IU/L) and alanine aminotransferase (ALT) concentration of 190 IU/L (normal range 10–50 IU/L). *What would you do next?*

Table 2
Common drug combinations containing acetaminophen (AMP). Current recommendations limit a 24-hour AMP dose to 4 g or less

Drug Name	Hydrocodone (mg)	AMP (mg)	Codeine (mg)
Lorcet	10	650	
Lortab (Vicodin)	5	500	
Lortab 7.5	7.5	500	
Lortab 10	10	500	
Norco	5	325	
Norco	7.5	325	
Norco	10	325	
Tylenol #3	–	300	30
Tylox	5 mg (oxycodone)	500	
Percocet	5 mg (oxycodone)	325	
Percocet	10 mg (oxycodone)	650	

The 60-year-old patient described in this section was switched from Lorcet to Norco.

Acetaminophen Toxicity

Prompt recognition of acetaminophen (acetyl-*para*-aminophenol [APAP], or, for this discussion, AMP) hepatotoxicity is key to preventing morbidity and mortality. With correct dosing, 90% of AMP is conjugated with glucuronide to form nontoxic metabolites. Approximately 5% of AMP is metabolized by the hepatic cytochrome p450 oxidase enzymes to a toxic metabolite, N-acetyl-p-benzoquinoneimine (NAPQI). In normal dosing, NAPQI is rapidly detoxified by glutathione (GSH) to nontoxic metabolites. Chronic AMP overdoses eventually overwhelm conjugation, and increased formation of NAPQI together with GSH depletion ultimately causes hepatic necrosis. Because alcohol (ethanol) induces the p450 enzyme system, the liver has increased capability to metabolize AMP to NAPQI. Chronic alcoholics also have lower plasma GSH levels than nonalcoholics, explaining reports of a significantly greater risk of developing hepatic necrosis in the alcoholic following chronic AMP ingestion. GSH is essential for the detoxification of NAPQI and GSH stores are also reported to be depleted by malnutrition and anorexia nervosa.[31] The Rumack-Matthew treatment (with N-acetylcysteine [NAC]) nomogram is useful in guiding treatment of acute AMP toxicity only, not for the subacute or chronic ingestion-induced toxicity that occurs in patients with chronic pain.

Subacute (chronic) AMP ingestions that result in hepatotoxicity occur in persons taking supratherapeutic doses of AMP and who are at increased risk for AMP-induced hepatotoxicity.[32] Serum concentrations of AMP, AST, and ALT should be measured in any patient at increased risk for hepatotoxicty (hepatitis, malnutrition, alcoholic, and so forth) who ingests more than 4 g of AMP per day. Patients with any AMP detected or with increased AST and ALT levels should be treated with oral NAC. Studies have shown that no patient with chronic AMP ingestion with an AST level less than 50 IU proceeded to develop hepatotoxicty, whereas 15% of those with an AST level greater than 50 IU did develop hepatotoxicty. Therefore, the patient described at the start of this section was treated with oral NAC and a change in his oral analgesic therapy (see **Table 2**).

Hepatotoxicty caused by AMP ingestion is believed to be effectively treated by NAC because NAC is a precursor for, and increases the synthesis of, GSH.[33] NAPQI will bind to the thiol groups of GSH instead of binding to hepatocytes. Once NAPQI is bound to the thiol group of GSH, it produces cysteine and mercapturic acid conjugates which are nonreactive with hepatocytes. A 72-hour oral NAC protocol is considered standard treatment of chronic AMP toxicity.[34]

Fentanyl Patches and Lollipops

The licit and illicit use of the continuous release fentanyl transdermal patch and the fentanyl lollipop has dramatically increased in the past decade.[35] Transdermal fentanyl patches are designed to release 12.5, 25, 50, 75, or 100 μg/h, and result in plasma levels of fentanyl similar to those achieved with a continuous IV infusion. The manufacturer recommends that the patches be replaced after 72 hours of continual use, at which time substantial amounts of fentanyl remain in the patch (approximately 2800 μg in a 10 mg patch). Because of the continued presence of fentanyl in used patches, the used patches have been smoked, ingested, the contents extracted and injected, and steeped in hot water (creating a fentanyl tea).[36] Abuse of the extracted fentanyl remaining in the reservoir results in an unreliable and unpredictable dose and has resulted in several overdose fatalities.[37]

The fentanyl lollipop (Actiq) depends on transmucosal absorption and is used primarily for cancer breakthrough pain. Abuse of either preparation of fentanyl presents the clinician with the well-known symptoms of opioid intoxication (CNS and respiratory depression, miosis) and is treated with standard supportive care and airway management.

DMP

DMP is the dextrorotatory isomer of levorphanol, a codeine analog, and is used primarily as a cough suppressant.[38] Widely available in various over-the-counter cough and cold preparations, DMP is found in Robitussin and Coricidin. Despite initial classification as an opioid, DMP was believed to lack the potential for abuse or addiction. DMP does not induce the typical opioid effects of respiratory depression, miosis, or analgesia because DMP does not bind to and stimulate the k or μ opioid receptors. Because the primary active metabolite is dextrorphan, which binds to and inhibits the N-methyl-D-aspartate (NMDA) receptor (as does DMP itself, a pharmacologic effect similar to that of ketamine), DMP abuse will produce the well-known phencyclidine (PCP)-like effects of visual hallucinations, euphoria, paranoia, disorientation, altered time perception, and acute psychosis.[39] In addition, DMP is a serotonin reuptake inhibitor and therefore is capable of causing the central serotonergic effects described earlier. Benzodiazapines, like midazolam, are effective in preventing or treating the CNS effects of the PCP-like drugs, and therefore should be a drug of choice in the treatment of the DMP-abusing patient.

POISONINGS CAUSING METABOLIC ACIDOSIS, INCLUDING CARBON MONOXIDE

A 3-year-old 16-kg boy presents to the emergency department following a mobile-home fire caused by a propane heater requiring the fire department to remove the patient through a rear bedroom window. On arrival, the patient is somnolent and, with face mask oxygen supplementation, a standard pulse oximeter reads an Spo_2 of 97%. Several minutes following admission, the patient experiences a seizure and a successful endotracheal intubation is performed. ABG analysis reveals a Po_2 of 97 mm Hg, pco_2 of 33 mm Hg, pH 7.19, base deficit −13 mmol/L, HCO_3^- of 12 mmol/L, and lactate of 7 mmol/L. An estimated 18% body surface area burn is localized to the lower extremity. *What would you do next?*

A toxin-induced metabolic acidosis (pH<7.40, reduced HCO_3^-, and the presence of a base deficit) can arise from increased acid production or impaired acid elimination. Increased acid production may be caused by toxins that are acidic or have acidic metabolites, cause the generation of ketoacid bodies, or interfere with adenosine triphosphate (ATP) production or consumption. Laboratory evaluation of these patients becomes essential, including quantitative testing for drugs (acetaminophen, aspirin, carboxyhemoglobin [CO-Hgb], ethylene glycol, and methanol), ABG analysis, metabolic panel studies, and 12-lead ECG. In addition, the patient may have clinical symptoms suggestive of well-described toxic syndromes caused by anticholinergic or cholinergic drugs, opioids, or sympathomimetic drugs. Routine serum and urine drug screens are seldom helpful, because the presence of a particular drug only confirms exposure to that drug, whereas that drug may not be the cause of the patient's clinical condition.

A clinically useful technique in the evaluation of a toxin-induced metabolic acidosis is the calculation of the anion gap (AG).[40] Many toxins are associated with an increased AG metabolic acidosis and the presence of an increased AG acidosis may suggest poisonings caused by several toxins (**Table 3**) and, in addition, may have prognostic value.[41] The AG is measured by the following formula: AG = $[Na^+]-[Cl^-]+[HCO_3^-]$. A normal AG is reported to be between 7 and 12 mEq/L,

Table 3
Medical conditions, toxins, or drugs that may cause increased AG metabolic acidosis

Medical Conditions	Toxin or Drugs
Uremia	Ethylene glycol
Diabetic ketoacidosis, alcoholic ketoacidosis	Salicylates
Lactic acidosis states, including shock	Acetaminophen
Carbon monoxide	Amphetamines Cocaine Cyanide (including nitroprusside) Metformin/phenformin Valproic acid Propofol

depending on the reference source chosen.[42] Thus a calculated AG greater than 12 mEq/L (±4 mEq/L) may suggest poisoning by one of the toxins or medical conditions listed in **Table 3**.

Acidosis Caused by Toxins that are Acids or Have Acid Metabolites (Increased Acid Production)

The alcohols benzyl alcohol, ethanol, ethylene glycol, and methanol are not acidifying per se until metabolized to acidic intermediates.[43] Ethylene glycol is metabolized to glycolic acid, methanol to formic acid, and ethanol to acetic acid. Benzyl alcohol is a common preservative in IV medications. Salicylates are weak acids that may produce an increased AG metabolic acidosis through several mechanisms, including the uncoupling of oxidative phosphorylation, renal injury leading to renal failure and acid retention, and cause an increase in acidic ketone body formation.[44]

Acidosis Caused by Toxin Interference with ATP Production or Consumption

Metabolic acidosis may result from disruption of cellular energy production or consumption. Acetaminophen is believed to inhibit (uncouple) oxidative phosphorylation that leads to an AG metabolic acidosis. Human immunodeficiency virus (HIV)-positive patients taking antiretroviral therapy may develop lactic acidosis by uncoupling oxidative phosphorylation via the inhibition of mitochondrial DNA polymerase. Increased AG metabolic acidosis is also a known result of valproic acid toxicity. The biguanide phenformin was withdrawn from clinical use because of the risk of metabolic acidosis. Another biguanide, metformin, has not to date been directly linked to metabolic acidosis, but an intentional overdose of metformin may cause AG metabolic acidosis by inhibition of the electron transport chain.[45]

Several mitochondrial poisons may cause profound metabolic acidosis, including carbon monoxide, cyanide (including nitroprusside-derived cyanide ion), formic acid (formed by the metabolism of ingested methanol), and salicylates. These toxins inhibit the electron transport chain, blocking aerobic energy production that may result in an increased AG metabolic acidosis.

Acidosis Caused by Increased Acid Production

Uncontrolled diabetes, prolonged fasting and exercise, and acute alcohol consumption can induce the production of ketone bodies (acetoacetate, acetone, β-hydroxybutyrate), resulting in an AG metabolic acidosis.

The presence of lactate is primarily an indicator of (or result of) anaerobic metabolism. No net increase in H^+ ion production occurs during the anaerobic metabolism of glucose to lactate in the production of ATP.[46] Other evidence supporting the understanding that lactate per se does not cause an AG metabolic acidosis is the observation that infusion of lactate containing fluids (Ringer lactate) results in an increase in pH because of liver metabolism of lactate to HCO_3^- and the frequent observation of increased AG metabolic acidosis in patients with normal lactate levels.[47]

Treatment of Metabolic Acidosis

It is important for the clinician to correctly diagnose and treat the underlying cause of an AG metabolic acidosis. Treating metabolic acidosis with a buffer like sodium bicarbonate has been shown to be injurious because of exacerbation of acidosis. Sodium bicarbonate therapy results in an increase in the generation of carbon dioxide, which has been shown to further lower pH, thereby exacerbating acidosis.[48] Currently, sodium bicarbonate should be viewed as a sodium ion donor, useful in antagonizing drug-induced sodium channel blockade found in clinical conditions like cocaine intoxication,[6] tricyclic antidepressant overdose, or LA toxicity; conditions characterized by a drug-induced sodium channel blockade. Patients who also may benefit from bicarbonate therapy are those poisoned with drugs whose elimination may be increased by alkalinization (salicylates).

Carbon Monoxide Poisoning

Carbon monoxide (CO) is the leading cause of poisoning deaths in the United States. A cigarette smoker is exposed to an estimated 400 to 500 ppm of CO while actively smoking. Exposure to 70 ppm may cause CO-Hgb levels to reach as high as 10% at equilibrium (4 hours). CO binds to Hgb with an affinity 200 times that of O_2, causing a leftward shift of the oxyhemoglobin dissociation curve. CO binds to many other heme-containing proteins other than Hgb, including cytochromes (impairing oxidative metabolism), myoglobin (skeletal and cardiac muscle toxicity), and guanylyl cyclase (increased nitric oxide [NO] levels).[49] Increased brain concentrations of NO are believed to play a major role in the neurologic injury following CO poisoning.

These pharmacologic effects of CO explain the diverse consequences of CO poisoning on the CNS (headache, confusion, seizure, and coma), heart (dysrhythmia, ischemia, infarction, asystole), and skeletal muscle (rhabdomyolysis and acute renal failure).

Delayed (2–40 days postpoisoning) neurologic deterioration following apparent recovery following CO poisoning is well described. This delayed deterioration is more common in those patients initially presenting in CO-induced coma.

A nonsmoker normally has 1% to 3% CO-Hgb, whereas smokers may have up to 10%. Low CO-Hgb levels (<15%) cause mild symptoms (nausea, headache), whereas levels of 60% to 70% are usually fatal. CO-Hgb levels should be measured with a CO-oximeter, which can accurately measure CO-Hgb and other abnormal hemoglobins (MHgb). Barker and Tremper[50] showed that Spo_2 measured by standard pulse oximetry (2 wavelengths) consistently overestimated o_2 saturation in the presence of CO-Hgb. Their data show that, at 70% CO-Hgb (usually fatal in humans), a standard 2-wavelength pulse oximeter Spo_2 read 90% saturation, whereas actual oxyhemoglobin levels were 30%. Their demonstration of a linear decrease of oxyhemoglobin with increasing CO-Hgb concentrations underscores the important role of CO-oximeter (multiple wavelength) monitoring in these patients.[50]

The severity of metabolic acidosis correlates with exposure duration, expression of clinical symptoms, and adverse outcomes following CO intoxication. The amount of lactate present serves as a marker for severe CO poisoning by reflecting the degree of anaerobic metabolism.

Treatment of CO poisoning begins with airway management, oxygen supplementation, and cardiovascular support. Hyperbaric oxygen therapy may have a role in preventing adverse neurologic outcomes but introduces unique problems and possible complications. Hyperbaric O_2 reduces the half-life of CO-Hgb: the half-life of CO-Hgb is 320 minutes with room air (21% O_2), 40 to 80 minutes at 100% O_2, and 20 minutes at 100% O_2 at 2.5 to 3 atmospheres.[51] In addition to reducing CO-Hgb concentrations, hyperbaric O_2 also reduces CO binding at all heme-containing protein sites (cytochromes, myoglobin, and so forth). Reports of reduction in the incidence of the delayed neurologic deterioration syndrome following CO poisoning makes the use of hyperbaric oxygen compelling for those patients whose presenting symptoms include coma.

High levels of CO-Hgb (36%) have been described during desflurane anesthesia in the presence of a dehydrated CO_2 absorbant (Baralyme).[52] Carbon dioxide absorbants containing strong alkali hydroxides (KOH, NaOH) are believed to be responsible for the degradation of inhaled anesthetic agents. The elimination of these strong alkali–containing absorbants have made CO_2 absorbent use safer, with minimal CO production with desflurane and isoflurane.[53] CO can also be formed during sevoflurane administration,[54] especially with Baralyme use. Because further studies are required to evaluate newer NaOH- and KOH-free absorbents, the need to avoid using dry CO_2 absorbent by frequent and routine servicing of the anesthesia machine remains, particularly in a location where patients with prior CO exposure may be anesthetized (the burn room).

The patient described at the start of this section had a measured CO-Hgb of 27%. He was treated with mechanical ventilation with high inspired oxygen concentrations and, as expected, within 12 hours the CO-Hgb concentration fell to less than 5%, allowing removal from mechanical ventilation and uneventful extubation.

MILITARY/TERRORIST POISONINGS, INCLUDING BOTULISM AND BOTOX

A 12-year-old boy is schedule for elective surgery requiring general anesthesia. He has a history of spastic cerebral palsy and was treated for the spasticity with injections of botulinum toxin type A (Botox) on 4 occasions (the most recent 2 weeks before) in the previous 18 months. How should this patient be anesthetized? If neuromuscular blocker (NMB) use is required, which one should be used and should a normal response be expected? Is NMB monitoring important in the management of this patient? Where should the effects of the NMB be monitored: at the eye brow (orbicularis oculi) or the hand (adductor pollicis), and would it make a difference clinically? *What would you do?*

Increasing attempts by terrorist organizations to manufacture weapons causing mass injuries and fatalities requires the clinician to have some awareness of the management of these injuries. Documented use of mustard gas and the nerve agent tabun by the Iraqi military during the Iran-Iraq war and production capabilities found for *Bacillus anthracis*, rotavirus, aflatoxin, mycotoxins, and botulinum toxin found following the Gulf War demonstrate the current danger facing modern society.

Initial management of the victims of chemical and biological weapons (CBWs) includes decontamination procedures (removal or neutralization of CBWs) to limit further exposure, such as showering and the use of chemical agents (soap, hypochlorite solutions), are important measures. Medical staff training in the use of protective equipment, including full-face mask, air-purifying equipment, and chemically resistant clothing and boots is essential.

Chemical Agents

Nerve agents (sarin, tabun, soman, VX) are toxic, odorless, colorless, and tasteless, are chemically related to the organophosphate insecticides, and are irreversible inhibitors of acetylcholinesterase (AChE).[55] Organophosphate insecticide (malathion) poisonings cause several hundred thousand fatalities worldwide every year. The cholinergic crisis syndrome resulting from the systemic overdose of acetylcholine (ACH) secondary to AChE inhibition results in the well-known symptoms of salivation, bronchospasm, skeletal muscle weakness/paralysis, bradycardia, and respiratory failure. The use of succinylcholine for neuromuscular blockade will result in prolonged paralysis because of the concomitant inhibition of the plasma cholinesterases. The first phase of the cholinergic crisis is characterized by a depolarizing block at the neuromuscular junction, whereas the second phase of muscle weakness is caused by a nondepolarizing (phase 2) block, all resulting from an overdose of ACH at the neuromuscular junction. Pyridostigmine has been recommended as a pretreatment because the inhibition of AChE is competitive and reversible. Atropine and the oximes (pralidoxime, which reactivates AChE) are effective if given early following exposure. Atropine is more effective that glycopyrrolate, which has a shorter half-life and does not cross the blood-brain barrier.

Blistering agents (the mustards, such as mustard gas and nitrogen mustard, and lewisite) are liquids that cause chemical burns and blisters, resulting in respiratory failure, blindness, pancytopenia, and cancer.[56] Mustard gas smells like mustard or garlic and can be released atmospherically by explosive aerosolization. Following a latent period of 4 to 12 hours, skin erythema appears on exposed areas, with edema and first-degree burns following. With high-dose exposure, skin necrosis and sloughing occurs, requiring treatment similar to burn therapy (fluid rescue, debridment). Ocular symptoms are common (pain, blurred vision) and may lead to permanent blindness. Inhalation of mustard gas causes tracheobronchitis, cough, bronchospasm, pulmonary hemorrhage, secondary bacterial lung infections, and respiratory failure that may require intubation and mechanical ventilation.

Choking agents (chlorine, phosgene, chloropicrin) are volatile liquids that cause fulminant pulmonary edema.[57] Chlorine and phosgene are widely used in the synthesis of plastics, and therefore poisoning with these agents may be encountered following industrial accidents. Phosgene smells like freshly mown hay, is hydrolyzed to CO_2 and hydrochloric acid, explaining phosgene's ability to cause severe lung injury (pulmonary edema) following inhalation. Treatment will include corticosteroids (inhaled or IV), inhaled β2 agonists, prophylactic antibiotics (for secondary bacterial infections), leukotriene inhibitors.

The blood agents hydrogen cyanide and cyanogen chloride inhibit the cytochrome oxidase system, causing a metabolic acidosis and tissue hypoxia resulting in seizures and respiratory and cardiac failure.[58] Hydrogen cyanide has an almond smell, is colorless, and rapidly fatal. Cyanide binds to the trivalent iron of cytochrome oxidase, interrupting the consumption of O_2. ABG analysis demonstrates an increased lactate (AG) metabolic acidosis and a reduced oxygen gradient between arterial and mixed venous blood, a characteristic finding in cyanide poisoning. Sodium thiosulfate, sodium nitrite, and hydroxycobalamin are effective treatment options.

Biologic Agents

All biologic agents have similar characteristics: release into an unprotected population with poor natural immunity will produce a high fatality and incapacitance rate. Biological weapons include viruses (variola), rickettsiae (Q fever, Rocky Mountain spotted fever), and bacteria [*B anthracis* (anthrax), *Yersinia pestis* (plague) and *Francisella tularensis* (tularemia)]. *Y pestis* in an anaerobic gram-negative coccobacillus and is transmitted to humans primarily by rodent fleas or human-to-human droplet infection. The clinical symptoms include pneumonia, fever, hemoptysis, sepsis, and multiple organ failure requiring ventilatory and circulatory support. Streptomycin, gentamicin, and chloramphenicol are effective for *Y pestis* eradication, whereas chemoprophylaxis is provided by tetracycline or doxycycline.

B anthracis is an aerobic, gram-positive spore-forming rod that primarily infects cattle, sheep, goats, and horses. Fifty kilograms of aerosolized *B anthracis* released upwind of half a million unprotected humans would kill an estimated 20%.[59] The most common clinical presentation is cutaneous anthrax, whereas inhalation of anthrax spores can result in a highly lethal form of the disease. The recent release of anthrax spores via the US mail system resulted in the cutaneous and inhalational expression of the disease. The inhalation form begins with a cough and fever and can progress to a necrotizing mediastinitis and multiple organ failure that is refractory to treatment and is usually fatal. An enzyme-linked immunosorbent assay (ELISA) is able to rapidly detect circulating toxin, whereas Gram stains and blood cultures are aids to a correct diagnosis. Ciprofloxacin and doxycycline may be used for chemoprophylaxis.

Saxitoxin, ricin, and botulinum toxin are the most toxic chemicals currently known, and they injure by a variety of mechanisms. *Clostridium botulinum* strains produce several neurotoxins that are the most toxic chemicals known. Neurotoxin A (Botox) binds to presynaptic ACH receptors, permanently inhibiting ACH release,[60] and requires the generation of new end-plate boutons to reestablish normal neuromuscular function.[61] Following botulinum toxin exposure, bulbar palsy (dysarthria, dysphagia, diplopia, ptosis) followed by progressive descending weakness ending in respiratory failure occurs, requiring prolonged mechanical ventilation for survival.

Ricin is derived from castor bean seeds and is a waste product of castor oil production. Inhalation of high doses is rapidly fatal, with no definitive treatment available. Saxitoxin is produced by a flagellate sea organism that produces the red tide. It can become concentrated in shellfish and is responsible for paralytic shellfish poisoning. Saxitoxin is a potent blocker of sodium channels, thereby resulting in a generalized failure of the cardiorespiratory system.

Humans who have received recent Botox therapy (such as the case described at the start of this section) may have an atypical response to NMBs. Fiacchino and colleagues[62] described resistance to a nondepolarizing NMB (vecuronium) in humans treated chronically with Botox and the mechanism is believed to be caused by a Botox-induced ACH receptor upregulation, similar to that seen following burn injury. There is a report describing the unmasking of occult myasthenia gravis shortly (first few days) following Botox injection. This report suggests a biphasic effect of Botox; that is, an early partial systemic neuromuscular blockade following the injection, implying an increased sensitivity to nondepolarizing NMBs could be expected to occur following recent (within a few days) Botox treatment.[63] The location of NMB monitoring may be particularly important in the patient treated with Botox because recovery studies evaluating respiratory (diaphragm) mechanics show that adequate recovery of airway protection and ventilatory adequacy may not occur until nearly complete neuromuscular recovery occurs, as demonstrated by adductor pollicis train-of-four ratio recovery of 0.80 or more.[64] Thus, monitoring the effect of NMBs at the adductor pollicis more accurately demonstrates complete diaphragm recovery and is therefore a more reliable margin of safety indicator-monitoring site compared with monitoring at the orbicularis occuli muscle.

POISONOUS BITES AND ENVENOMATIONS

An 8-year-old boy weighing 30 kg presents to the emergency room after sustaining a bite (confirmed by fang marks) to the right lower leg by the southern copperhead (*Agkistrodon contortrix*). The leg is currently swollen and edematous, indicating severe envenomation. Antivenin therapy was started (following negative skin tests), but the patient did not receive the full calculated dose because of urticaria, bronchospasm, and wheezing. Following treatment with histamine blockers and epinephrine, the patient developed what appeared to be an anterior compartment syndrome, confirmed by measured compartment pressures greater than 40 mm Hg. The patient is now scheduled for an emergency fasciotomy. What further laboratory tests, including tests for a possible coagulation disorder, should be ordered before proceeding with anesthesia? Does this history influence the choice for NMBs? Would an altered response to NMBs be expected? Would regional anesthesia (spinal or epidural) have a place in the anesthetic management of this patient? *How would you proceed?*

Marine Envenomations

Invertebrate envenomations include jellyfish (schyphozoa), anemones, and fire coral (hydrozoa). The most dangerous of the hydrozoas is the Portuguese man-of-war which can be found in the Atlantic Ocean and Gulf of Mexico and can cause fatal envenomations. In Australia, the jellyfish species *Carukia barnesi* can cause severe and sometimes fatal envenomations.[65] The symptoms of envenomations include muscle cramps and headache, which may progress to hypertension, pulmonary and cerebral edema, and cardiac failure. Jellyfish venoms are antigenic, causing a variety of reactions, including rash, skin necrosis, neural and cardiac toxicity, and hemolysis. Death has resulted from anaphylaxis, but other symptoms include nausea, vomiting, headache, confusion, seizures, muscle spasm, angioedema with airway loss, and severe bronchospasm. Treatment includes flooding the envenomation site with 5% acetic acid (household vinegar), whereas isopropyl alcohol will cause further discharge of unfired nematocysts and is not recommended.[66] IV magnesium sulfate reduces pain[67] and the sympathetic response to envenomation; hot water (43–45°C) immersion, including total body shower with hot water following widespread envenomation, will inactivate the venom.

The echinoderm most commonly involved in envenomation is the sea urchin. The usual presentation is envenomation following a human stepping on the sea urchin, breaking off venom-containing spines into the skin. Treatment is similar to that of jellyfish envenomation.

Vertebrate envenomations include stingrays, lionfish, and stonefish. Stingray envenomation is the most common.[68] Although potentially serious cardiac dysrhythmias, seizures, and coma have been reported, the more likely life-threatening injuries are puncture wounds of the abdomen or chest. Wound irrigation followed by hot water immersion (causing venom degradation) is usually adequate treatment. Lionfish envenomation is characterized by severe localized pain and swelling. Treatment is the same as for stingray envenomation.[69] Antivenom is only available for stonefish envenomations.

Snake Envenomations

Two families of poisonous snakes are found in North America: the crotalids and elapids.

The crotalid (rattlesnake, cottonmouth, copperhead) are responsible for most envenomations.[70] The spectrum of clinical presentations from crotalid bites range from asymptomatic to cardiovascular collapse and death. Tissue damage at the bite site is the most common complication following envenomation. Hemorrhagic toxins cause damage to capillary endothelium, allowing red blood cell extravasation that causes edema and hemorrhagic blebs. Venom metalloproteinases cleave protumor necrosis factor (pro-TNF), releasing active TNF, which initiates an aggressive inflammatory response.[71] This aggressive inflammatory response makes an accurate diagnosis of compartment syndrome difficult, requiring objective measurement of compartment pressures a requirement for correct diagnosis. A clinical coagulopathy is found in up to 50% of bite victims.[72] Venom may cause lysis of fibrinogen and fibrin leading to complete defibrination and platelet aggregation leading to widespread thrombosis and thrombocytopenia. Therefore, regional anesthesia should be approached with extreme caution in the bite victim. Neuromuscular blockade secondary to calcium channel blockade that inhibits ACH release is known to occur, especially with the Mojave rattlesnake (*Crotalus scutulatus*, commonly found in the American southwest),[73] and potentially synergize with NMBs.

Treatment depends on the severity of the envenomation. With extremity swelling, compartment syndrome must be documented with pressure measurement (>30 mm Hg) before fasciotomy.[74] Antivenom is the treatment of choice for crotalid bite–induced coagulopathy. Two antivenom products are available: a polyvalent antivenom of equine origin, and an ovine (sheep) polyvalent Fab immunoglobulin fragment product. Hypersensitivity to the equine product makes the sheep-derived product the preferred antivenom. Padda and Bowen[75] published a case report on rapid onset and prolonged duration of a nondepolarizing neuromuscular blocking agent (vecuronium) following human envenomation by a northern copperhead. Thus, for a recent envenomation victim, the administration of NMBs should be carefully titrated and adequate reversal documented by continuous neuromuscular monitoring by nerve stimulation.

SUMMARY

Drug- or toxin-induced pathology that the clinician may encounter and therapeutic approaches to these syndromes are discussed in this review. Although these syndromes have diverse causes and mechanisms of injury, they are organized by shared or similar mechanisms of injury and pathophysiology to present a more cohesive and understandable discussion.

REFERENCES

1. Wong KC, Schafer PG, Schultz JR. Hypokalemia and anesthetic implications. Anesth Analg 1993;77:1238–60.
2. Maruyama T, Ohe T, Kurita T, et al. Physiological and pathological responses of TU wave to class Ia antiarrhythmic drugs. Eur Heart J 1995;16:667–73.
3. Elming H, Brendorp B, Kober L, et al. QTc interval in the assessment of cardiac risk. Card Electrophysiol Rev 2002;6:289–94.
4. Haddad PM, Anderson IM. Antipsychotic-related QTc prolongation, torsade de pointes and sudden death. Drugs 2002;62:1649–71.
5. McCord J, Jneid H, Hollander JE, et al. Management of cocaine-associated chest pain and myocardial infarction. Circulation 2008;117:1897–907.
6. Beckman KJ, Parker RB, Hariman RJ, et al. Hemodynamic and electrophysiological actions of cocaine. Circulation 1991;83:1799–807.
7. Bauman JL, Grawe JJ, Winecoff AP, et al. Cocaine-related sudden cardiac death: a hypothesis correlating basic science and clinical observations. J Clin Pharmacol 1994;34:902–11.

8. Ehret GB, Voide C, Gex-Fabry M, et al. Drug-induced long QT syndrome in injection drug users receiving methadone. Arch Intern Med 2006;166: 1280–7.
9. Siebrands CC, Binder S, Eckhoff U, et al. Long QT 1 mutation KCNQ1 increases local anesthetic sensitivity of the slowly activating delayed rectifier potassium current. Anesthesiology 2006;105:511–20.
10. Park WK, Kim MH, Ahn DS, et al. Myocardial depressant effects of desflurane. Anesthesiology 2007;106:956–66.
11. Lischke V, Behne M, Doelken P, et al. Droperidol causes a dose-dependent prolongation of the QT interval. Anesth Analg 1994;79:983–6.
12. Darling RC, Roughton FJW. The effect of methemoglobin on the equilibrium between oxygen and hemoglobin. Am J Physiol 1942;137:56–68.
13. Bloom JC, Brandt JT. Toxic responses of the blood. In: Klaassen CD, editor. Casarett and Doull's toxicology: the basic science of poisons online. 6th edition. New York: McGraw-Hill; 2001. p. 389–417, chapter 11.
14. Guay J. Methemoglobinemia related to local anesthetics: a summary of 242 episodes. Anesth Analg 2009;108:837–45.
15. Annabi EH, Barker SJ. Severe methemoglobinemia detected by pulse oximetry. Anesth Analg 2009;108:898–9.
16. Harley JD, Celermajer JM. Neonatal methemoglobin anemia and the "red-brown" screening test. Lancet 1970;296:1223–5.
17. Barker SJ, Tremper KK. Effects of methemoglobinemia on pulse oximetry and mixed venous oximetry. Anesthesiology 1989;70:112–7.
18. FDA MedWatch-Public Health Advisory Bulletin re: benzocaine spray and methemoglobinemia, February 13, 2006.
19. Steele CW, Spink WW. Methylene blue in the treatment of poisonings associated with methemoglobinemia. N Engl J Med 1933;208:1152–3.
20. Bodner RA, Lynch T, Lewis L, et al. Serotonin syndrome. Neurology 1995;45: 219–23.
21. Asch DA, Parker RM. The Libby Zion case. One step forward or two steps backward? N Engl J Med 1988;318:771–5.
22. Mills KC. Serotonin syndrome. A clinical update. Crit Care Clin 1997;13:763–83.
23. Miller DB, O'Callaghan JP. Elevated environmental temperature and methamphetamine neurotoxicity. Environ Res 2003;92:48–53.
24. Sprague JE, Moze P, Caden D, et al. Carvedilol reverses hyperthermia and attenuates rhabdomyolysis induced by 3,4-methylenedioxymethamphetamine (MDMA, Ecstasy) in an animal model. Crit Care Med 2005;33:1311–6.
25. Friedman LS, Weinrauch LA, D'Elia JP. Metoclopramide-induced neuroleptic malignant syndrome. Arch Intern Med 1987;147:1495–7.
26. Andersson B, Waagstein F. Spectrum and outcome of congestive heart failure in a hospitalized population. Am Heart J 1993;126(3 Pt 1):632–40.
27. Koskinen P, Kupari M, Leinonen H, et al. Alcohol and new onset atrial fibrillation: a case-control study of a current series. Br Heart J 1987;57:468–73.
28. Gurley BJ, Wang P, Gardner SF. Ephedrine-type alkaloid content of nutritional supplements containing *Ephedra sinica* (ma-huang) as determined by high performance liquid chromatography. J Pharm Sci 1998;87:1547–53.
29. Haller CA, Benowitz NL. Adverse cardiovascular and central nervous system events associated with dietary supplements containing ephedra alkaloids. N Engl J Med 2000;343:1833–8.
30. Vormfelde SV, Poser W. Hyperforin in extracts of St. John's wort (*Hypericum perforatum*) for depression. Arch Intern Med 2000;160:2548–9.

31. Rumack BH. Acetaminophen hepatotoxicity: the first 35 years. J Toxicol Clin Toxicol 2002;40:3–20.
32. Daly FF, O'Malley GF, Heard K, et al. Prospective evaluation of repeated supratherapeutic acetaminophen (paracetamol) ingestion. Ann Emerg Med 2004;44: 393–8.
33. Bajt ML, Knight TR, Lemasters JJ, et al. Acetaminophen-induced oxidant stress and cell injury in cultured mouse hepatocytes: protection by N-acetyl cysteine. Toxicol Sci 2004;80:343–9.
34. Taylor SE. Acetaminophen intoxication and length of treatment: how long is long enough? A comment. Pharmacotherapy 2004;24:694–6 [discussion: 696].
35. Purucker M, Swann W. Potential for duragesic patch abuse. Ann Emerg Med 2000;35:314.
36. Barrueto FJ. The fentanyl tea bag. Vet Hum Toxicol 2004;46:30–1.
37. Reeves MD, Ginifer CJ. Fatal intravenous misuse of transdermal fentanyl. Med J Aust 2002;177:552–3.
38. Bern JL, Peck R. Dextromethorphan: an overview of safety issues. Drug Saf 1992; 7:190–9.
39. Price L, Lebel J. Dextromethorphan-induced psychosis. Am J Psychiatry 2000; 157:304.
40. Salem MM, Mujais SK. Gaps in the anion gap. Arch Intern Med 1992;152:1625–9.
41. Brenner BE. Clinical significance of the elevated anion gap. Am J Med 1985;79: 289–96.
42. Ishihara K, Szerlip HM. Anion gap acidosis. Semin Nephrol 1998;18:83–97.
43. Gabow PA, Clay K, Sullivan JB, et al. Organic acids in ethylene glycol intoxication. Ann Intern Med 1986;105:16–20.
44. Alberti KG, Cohen RD, Woods HF. Lactic acidosis and hyperlactataemia. Lancet 1974;2:1519–60.
45. Salpeter SR, Greyber E, Pasternak GA, et al. Risk of fatal and nonfatal lactic acidosis with metformin use in type 2 diabetes mellitus: systematic review and meta-analysis. Arch Intern Med 2003;163:2594–602.
46. Stacpoole PW. Lactic acidosis. Endocrinol Metab Clin North Am 1993;22:221–45.
47. Gabow PA, Kaehny WD, Fennessey PV, et al. Diagnostic importance of an increased serum anion gap. N Engl J Med 1980;303:854–8.
48. Adrogue HJ, Rashad MN, Gorin AB, et al. Assessing acid-base status in circulatory failure. N Engl J Med 1989;320:1312–6.
49. Brown SD, Piantadosi CA. Reversal of carbon monoxide-cytochrome c oxidase binding by hyperbaric oxygen in vivo. Adv Exp Med Biol 1989;248:747–54.
50. Barker SJ, Tremper KK. The effect of carbon monoxide inhalation on pulse oximetry and transcutaneous po_2. Anesthesiology 1987;66:677–9.
51. Jay GD, McKindley DS. Alterations in pharmacokinetics of carboxyhemoglobin produced by oxygen under pressure. Undersea Hyperb Med 1997;24:165–73.
52. Berry PD, Sessler DI, Larson MD. Severe carbon monoxide poisoning during desflurane anesthesia. Anesthesiology 1999;90:613–6.
53. Kharasch ED, Powers KM, Artru AA. Comparison of Amsorb, Soda lime and Baralyme. Degradation of volatile anesthetics and formation of carbon monoxide and compound A in swine in vivo. Anesthesiology 2002;96:173–82.
54. Holak EJ, Mei DA, Dunning MB, et al. Carbon monoxide production from sevoflurane breakdown: modeling of exposures under clinical conditions. Anesth Analg 2003;96:757–64.
55. Karalliedde L. Organophosphorus poisoning and anaesthesia. Anaesthesia 1999;54:1073–88.

56. Borak MD, Sidell FR. Agents of chemical warfare: sulfur mustard. Ann Emerg Med 1992;21:303-8.
57. Brennan RJ, Waeckerle JF, Sharp TW, et al. Chemical warfare agents: emergency medical and emergency public health issues. Ann Emerg Med 1999;34:191-204.
58. Baskin SI, Brewer TG. Cyanide poisoning. In: Zajtchuk R, editor. Textbook of military medicine: medical aspects of chemical and biological warfare. Washington, DC: US Department of the Army; 1997. p. 271-86.
59. Kaufmann AF, Meltzer MI, Schmid GP. The economic impact of a bioterrorist attack: are prevention and past attack programs justifiable? Emerg Infect Dis 1997;3:83-94.
60. Moles TM, Baker DJ. Clinical analogies for the management of toxic trauma. Resuscitation 1999;42:125-31.
61. Pasricha PJ, Ravich WJ, Kalloo AN. Effects of intrasphincteric botulinum toxin on the lower esophageal sphincter in piglets. Gastroenterology 1993;105:1045-9.
62. Fiacchino F, Grandi L, Soliveri P, et al. Sensitivity to vecuronium after botulinum toxin administration. J Neurosurg Anesthesiol 1997;9:149-53.
63. Ergbuth F, Claus D, Engelhardt A, et al. Systemic effects of local botulinum toxin injections unmasks subclinical Lambert-Eaton myasthenic syndrome. J Neurol Neurosurg Psychiatr 1993;56:1235-6.
64. Viby-Mogensen J, Engbaek J, Eriksson LI, et al. Good clinical research practice in pharmacodynamic studies of neuromuscular blocking agents. Acta Anaesthesiol Scand 1996;40:59-74.
65. Flecker H. "Irukandji" stings to north Queensland bathers without production of wheals but with severe general symptoms. Med J Aust 1952;2:89-91.
66. Nomura JT, Sato RL, Ahern RM, et al. A randomized paired comparison trial of cutaneous treatments for acute jellyfish (*Carybdea alata*) stings. Am J Emerg Med 2002;20:624-6.
67. Corkeron MA. Magnesium infusion to treat Irukandji syndrome. Med J Aust 2003; 178:411-2.
68. Auerbach PS. Envenomation by aquatic invertebrates. In: Auerback PS, editor. Wilderness medicine. 4th edition. St. Louis (MO): Mosby; 2001. p. 1488-95.
69. Kizer KW, McKinney HE, Auerbach PS. Scorpaenidae envenomation: a five-year poison center experience. JAMA 1985;253:807-10.
70. Watson WA, Litovitz TL, Klein-Schwartz W, et al. 2003 annual report of the American Association of Poison Control Centers Toxic Exposure Surveillance System. Am J Emerg Med 2004;22:335-404.
71. Laing GD, Clissa PB, Theakston RD, et al. Inflammatory pathogenesis of snake venom metalloproteinase-induced skin necrosis. Eur J Immunol 2003;33: 3458-63.
72. Cruz NS, Alvarez RG. Rattlesnake bite complications in 19 children. Pediatr Emerg Care 1994;10:30-3.
73. Valdes JJ, Thompson RRG, Wolff VL, et al. Inhibition of calcium channel dihydropyridine receptor binding by purified Mojave toxin. Neurotoxicol Teratol 1989;11: 129-33.
74. Mars M, Hadley GP, Aitchison JM. Direct intracompartmental pressure measurement in the management of snakebites in children. S Afr Med J 1991;80:227-8.
75. Padda GS, Bowen CH. Anesthetic implication of snake-bite envenomation. Anesth Analg 1995;81:649-51.

How to Manage Perioperative Endocrine Insufficiency

Benjamin A. Kohl, MD[a],*, Stanley Schwartz, MD[b]

KEYWORDS

- Endocrine • Perioperative • Diabetes • Hyperthyroidism
- Hypothyroidism • Adrenal insufficiency • Pheochromocytoma

Patients with endocrinopathies frequently present to the operating room. Although many of these disorders are managed on a chronic basis, patients may have acute changes in the perioperative period that, if left unrecognized, can have a negative effect on perioperative morbidity and mortality. It is imperative that anesthesiologists understand the implications of the surgical stress response on hormonal flux. This article focuses on the 4 most commonly encountered endocrinopathies: diabetes mellitus (DM), hyperthyroidism, hypothyroidism, and adrenal insufficiency. Specific challenges pertaining to patients with pheochromocytoma are also discussed.

DM

Diabetes is the most common endocrinopathy in the United States. Familiarity with its pathogenesis and management is therefore critical for perioperative clinicians. Approximately 90% of patients with DM are classified as type 2 and the remainder are type 1. It is estimated that more than 50% of this entire population will require surgery at some point during their lifetime.[1] From a resource utilization standpoint, the average patient with DM spends up to 50% more time in the hospital postoperatively than a patient without DM undergoing the same procedure.[2] Complications that are a direct result of this disease (neuropathy, retinopathy, nephropathy, and vasculopathy) often culminate in the need for surgery.

A version of this article originally appeared in the 93:5 issue of *Medical Clinics of North America*.

[a] Department of Anesthesiology and Critical Care, University of Pennsylvania School of Medicine, 3400 Spruce Street, Dulles Building, Suite 680, Philadelphia, PA 19104, USA
[b] Department of Medicine, Philadelphia Heart Institute, University of Pennsylvania Health System, 51 North 39th Street, Suite 400, Philadelphia, PA 19104, USA
* Corresponding author.
E-mail address: Benjamin.Kohl@uphs.upenn.edu

Anesthesiology Clin 28 (2010) 139–155
doi:10.1016/j.anclin.2010.01.003
1932-2275/10/$ – see front matter © 2010 Elsevier Inc. All rights reserved.

Type 1 DM (T1DM) is a consequence of the destruction and loss of pancreatic β cells (insulin producing). On the contrary, type 2 DM (T2DM) is a disease characterized by the interaction of genetic and environmental factors (stress, diet, and amount of exercise), culminating in insulin resistance, abnormal β-cell function and, ultimately, the development of overt T2DM. T2DM results when compensatory increases in insulin secretion can no longer keep plasma glucose levels within normal limits because of abnormal β-cell mass and function and inappropriate release of glucagon by pancreatic α cells.

Although these 2 classes effectively discriminate most patients with diabetes, it is important for the perioperative clinician to understand that other conditions may result in a similar phenotype, such as pancreatitis and pancreatic cancer. Patients destined to develop T2DM will have a prediabetic state of impaired glucose tolerance (IGT) diagnosed by a fasting blood glucose level greater than 100 mg/dL or 2-hour postprandial glucose level of 140 mg/dL or greater after a standard glucose challenge. This finding is critical as it has been shown that patients coming into hospital with previously unrecognized abnormal glucose tolerance, or overt DM, have worse outcomes and a greater number of complications during the hospitalization, often in association with surgical procedures.[3] Major efforts should be instituted to identify these patients before or on admission and criteria for those at special risk have recently been delineated.[4]

The ability of perioperative clinicians to risk stratify these patients appropriately and develop an interventional strategy depends on the individual patient, and the associated pathologic condition. Although anesthesiologists are rarely involved in the long-term care of these patients, the consequences of uncontrolled diabetes (ie, electrolyte imbalances, dehydration, wound infection) in the perioperative period can be life threatening.[5–8] Therefore, appropriate risk stratification and an optimal interventional strategy are necessary.

It is imperative to do a careful preoperative assessment for all patients as the patient with DM requires a systematic approach because the disease affects numerous organ systems (**Table 1**). Furthermore, although the surgical stress response is similar for a given procedure, patients with DM (particularly those with T1DM) are less able to counteract the effects of the gluconeogenic and glycolytic hormones (ie, cortisol, epinephrine, glucagon, growth hormone) that are released, all of which counteract the effect of insulin and may contribute to hyperglycemia.

Before examining the patient, there are several laboratory values that can help discern the severity of disease. Glycosylated hemoglobin (Hb_{A1C}) values can reflect the degree of hyperglycemia to which red blood cells (RBC) have been exposed. Because the average lifespan of an RBC is 120 days, the Hb_{A1C} is an indicator of glycemic levels over that period of time (although it is more strongly related to the prior 8–12 weeks). A normal value is up to 6%, but some patients with values greater than 5.5% may have IGT. The American Diabetes Association goal for DM control is less than 7%. Values more than 8% correspond to average blood glucose level of more than 180 mg/dL and indicate poor glycemic control.[9]

Because diabetes is a leading cause of renal failure, measurement of renal function can give insight into the severity of disease. Furthermore, of particular concern to the perioperative clinician, patients with DM with renal insufficiency are at greater risk for hypoglycemia given the prolonged half-life of insulin and sulfonylureas. By identifying these patients preoperatively, more frequent (every 30–60 minutes) monitoring of blood glucose may be anticipated. Although a serum creatinine value itself does not

Table 1
Perioperative considerations for complications and associated conditions of DM

Complications	Perioperative Considerations
Neuropathies	
Peripheral sensory	Heel pads, avoid heating pads
Cystopathy	Inability to urinate, overflow incontinence, urinary tract infections, consider straight catheterization
Gastroparesis	Watch for medications that slow gastric motility; reflux esophagitis/gastritis
Hypoglycemic unawareness	Frequent monitoring
Cardiovascular autonomic neuropathy	Arrhythmias: telemetry
Silent ischemia: angina without chest pain	Watch for unexplained dyspnea, hypotension, arrhythmias
Retinopathy	
Lens	Blurred vision with either worse control or with sudden improvement in chronic DM out of control
Proliferative retinopathy	Rule out preoperatively if no routine eye examination in past year
Nephropathy	Careful decision on use of intravenous iodinated contrast
Hyporenin, hypoaldosterone state	Watch for hyperkalemia Avoid hypotension
Macrophage dysfunction with blood sugar level greater than 150 mg/dL	Increased risk of infections; increased risk of fungal disease with parenteral nutrition Delayed would healing
Other conditions	
Hyperlipidemia	Statins valuable in hospital
Hypertension	Treat: watch potassium level, edema, pulse rate

diagnose renal impairment, in the steady state it gives a good estimate of glomerular filtration rate (GFR) via the Cockcroft-Gault equation[10]:

$$GFR = \frac{(140 - age) \times weight\ (kg) \times (0.85\ if\ female)}{72 \times serum\ creatinine}$$

Preoperative evaluation of patients with DM should focus on some of the more common association and sequelae of the disease process (**Table 1**). These patients are at increased risk for cerebrovascular accidents, myocardial infarctions, acute renal failure, and postoperative wound complications. This risk may be mitigated with control of perioperative hyperglycemia. Musculoskeletal manifestations are common and may predict difficulties with laryngoscopy and endotracheal intubation.[11] A positive prayer sign (inability to approximate fingers and palms with fingers extended) may be an indicator of joint rigidity.[12] Such complications are important to note in the perioperative period and provisions should be taken to minimize further exacerbation.

The major goals for these patients pertinent to their endocrinopathy should be minimizing hyperglycemia and avoiding hypoglycemia, hypovolemia, and hypo- or hyperkalemia. In addition, minimizing the length of time these patients remain nil by mouth is important. Surgery and anesthesia invoke a stress response in patients that is characterized by hypersecretion of counterregulatory hormones (eg, glucagon, norepinephrine, cortisol, and growth hormone). This response culminates in increased gluconeogenesis, glycogenolysis, and peripheral insulin resistance. Endogenous insulin levels are dramatically increased in the face of injury despite often profound hyperglycemia (ie, relative insulin deficiency). The effect of this altered hormonal milieu may culminate in diabetic ketoacidosis (DKA) in patients with T1DM and hyperosmolar hyperglycemic nonketosis in patients with T2DM.[13] Understanding this hormonal imbalance is fundamental to appreciating the fine endocrine balance these patients withstand in the perioperative period (**Fig. 1**). On the one hand, the surgical stress response initiates counterregulatory hormone secretion and relative insulin deficiency, culminating in hyperglycemia. On the other, perioperative fasting with increased endogenous and exogenous insulin can easily cause profound hypoglycemia. Thus, a perioperative strategy that anticipates this condition and aims to restore normoglycemia should be undertaken.

Although the approach to outpatient diabetic management is to aim for the lowest sugar possible without undue hypoglycemia, a similar perioperative goal is less realistic and potentially dangerous.[14,15] Although there are no current guidelines on perioperative glycemic control, the American College of Endocrinology has released a position statement on inpatient glycemic control.[16] Understanding that the perioperative period is unique, a reasonable approach would be to maintain blood glucose levels less than 200 mg/dL intraoperatively and less than 150 mg/dL postoperatively, but to avoid levels less than 80 mg/dL.[17,18] This strategy would avoid severe hyperglycemia and minimize hypoglycemia. Patients who are insulin dependent often require a change in their scheduled dosing dependent on how long they are nil by mouth before surgery, the frequency of their insulin administration, and when the case is scheduled (**Box 1**). Thiazoladinediones (TZD) can be held on the morning of surgery, and secretagogues must be held preoperatively. However, the biguanide metformin, which has been associated with the development of lactic acidosis, should be withheld 24 hours preoperatively and restarted 48 to 72 hours postoperatively once normal renal function has been

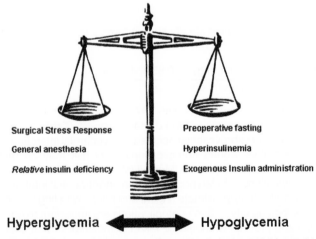

Hyperglycemia ⬅➡ Hypoglycemia

Surgical Stress Response | Preoperative fasting
General anesthesia | Hyperinsulinemia
Relative insulin deficiency | Exogenous Insulin administration

Fig. 1. The glycemic balance in the perioperative period. (*Adapted from* Kohl BA, Schwartz S. Surgery in the patient with endocrine dysfunction. Anesthesiol Clin 2009;27(4):687–703; with permission.)

Box 1
Perioperative management of insulin-dependent diabetes

- Need basal insulin at all times to avoid DKA

Night before procedure

- Continue usual dose of PM glargine/NPH or mixture (can recommend two-thirds usual dose if tightly controlled) the night before surgery (as long as taking usual by mouth intake the night before the operation)
- For insulin pump users: continue usual overnight basal rate

Morning of procedure

- No boluses of short-acting hypoglycemics unless blood sugar level is greater than 200 mg/dL and greater than 3 hours preoperative
- May place on insulin drip or give usual dose of glargine if routinely taken in morning
- For insulin pump users: continue usual basal rate and infuse D5 throughout operation
- If on NPH or other insulin mixture:
  - No short-acting insulin within 3 to 4 hours of procedure (ie, no mixture preoperatively)
  - Give half usual intermediate-acting insulin, with D5, at controlled rate throughout procedure
  - If performing operation without continuous D5, give no insulin preoperatively

Special situations

- Emergency surgery
  - No bolus of short-acting hypoglycemics preoperatively. Frequent (every 30–60 minutes) monitoring of blood sugar level throughout operation. Start insulin infusion if blood sugar level is greater than 200 mg/dL
- Cardiac surgery
  - Continue insulin infusion as needed to maintain blood glucose level at 100 to 150 mg/dL in first 3 postoperative days.

Abbreviations: D5, 5% dextrose containing solution; NPH, neutral protamine Hagedorn.
(*Adapted from* Kohl BA, Schwartz S. Surgery in the patient with endocrine dysfunction. Anesthesiol Clin 2009;27(4):687–703; with permission.)

---

documented.[19,20] Long-acting sulfonylureas (ie, chlorpropramide), although rarely used, are best withheld 48 to 72 hours preoperatively to avoid potential hypoglycemia.[21] Incretins may be given (incretin mimetics subcutaneously and dipeptidyl peptidase 4 inhibitors by mouth with a sip of water on the morning of surgery) because, in the absence of insulin or secretagogues, they do not cause hypoglycemia and seem particularly effective in reducing perioperative hyperglycemia as they counteract the effect of steroids on decreasing β-cell function, best demonstrated in a murine model.[22–24] Antihyperglycemic agents (TZDs and incretins) and secretagogues may be restarted once enteral intake is permitted, although metformin is commonly avoided postoperatively in the hospital in case intercurrent events ensue that might change renal function acutely (eg, hypotension, iodine dye–induced renal dysfunction, sepsis) and risk lactic acidosis. **Box 1** summarizes perioperative insulin therapy recommendations in those patients (T1DM and T2DM) who routinely require insulin. In general, all of these patients should be scheduled as first case of the day to minimize a significant endocrine imbalance.

There remains a paucity of data to guide the clinician on intraoperative glycemic control. The population that has been most heavily scrutinized has been cardiac surgery. There remains significant clinical equipoise regarding the potential benefit of tight intraoperative glycemic control even in this subset of patients.[25–30] However, although no formal recommendations have been made, most clinicians would agree that maintaining plasma glucose level less than 200 mg/dL intraoperatively is reasonable. Similar consensus exists for the noncardiac surgical population.[31]

Postoperatively, attempts should be made to initiate enteral intake as soon as possible. This process should be undertaken carefully, and in consultation with a nutritionist familiar with the needs of patients with diabetes.[32] Postoperative glycemic control has been (and continues to be) investigated thoroughly. Although there seems to be benefit with glycemic control in relation to postoperative surgical site infection,[5,33,34] there continues to be significant equipoise as this treatment modality relates to other morbidities and mortality.[35,36]

HYPERTHYROIDISM

The causes of hyperthyroidism are myriad. However, by far, the most common cause in the United States is Graves disease. This is an autoimmune disorder caused by antibody generation directed at thyroid-stimulating hormone (TSH) receptors, causing an increase in thyroid hormone production. Clinical signs and symptoms of hyperthyroidism include tachycardia, atrial fibrillation, fever, tremor, goiter, and ophthalmopathy. Other manifestations include gastrointestinal symptoms such as diarrhea, nausea, and emesis. Not all patients present with the classic symptomatology or laboratory findings. Patients with subclinical (masked) hyperthyroidism often are asymptomatic and frequently have normal free thyroid hormone levels with suppressed TSH. This entity is more common in the geriatric population. In clinically overt hyperthyroidism free thyroid hormone (T_4 and T_3) levels are frequently mildly increased; however, TSH is usually suppressed. In states of thyrotoxicosis, free T_4 levels can be dramatically increased. T_3 and T_4 have direct inotropic and chronotropic effects on the heart. In addition, thyroid hormones have a direct effect on vascular smooth muscle, causing a decrement in systemic vascular resistance and mean arterial blood pressure. As a result, the renin-angiotensin-aldosterone system is activated, enhancing sodium reabsorption and increasing circulating blood volume, increasing cardiac output by 50% to 300% (**Fig. 2**).[37,38] Chronically increased levels of these hormones may limit the ability of patients to respond to the stress of surgery and can culminate in cardiovascular collapse.[39–41] The perioperative clinician must be familiar with the diagnosis and treatment of hyperthyroidism as failure to identify and treat appropriately can drastically increase mortality.

Patients with hyperthyroidism should take their antithyroid medications on the morning of surgery.[42] For those patients with uncontrolled hyperthyroidism who are presenting for elective surgery, their surgical procedure should be postponed until they are on a stable medical regimen to reduce their risk of thyroid storm.[43] For those patients presenting for urgent or emergent surgery, it is incumbent on the anesthesiologist to have ready access to drugs that block the systemic effects of excess thyroid hormone. Such drugs include β-blockers, antithyroid medications (including propylthiouracil [PTU] and methimazole), and iodine. β-Blockers not only directly inhibit sympathetic activation but also inhibit the peripheral conversion of T_4 to T_3 (the most active thyroid hormone). Thionamides, such as PTU and methimazole, are actively transported into the thyroid gland and inhibit further production of hormone. Furthermore, PTU inhibits peripheral conversion of T_4 to T_3.[44] Inorganic iodide,

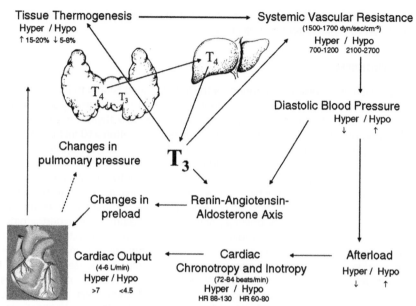

Fig. 2. Cardiovascular effects of thyroid hormone. (*From* Klein I, Danzi S. Thyroid disease and the heart. Circulation 2007;116:1725; with permission.)

although necessary for normal thyroid function, in excess manifests an antithyroid action known as the Wolff-Chaikoff effect.[45] Potassium iodide is given enterally as either Lugol solution (8 mg iodide per drop) or saturated solution of potassium iodide (SSKI) and is usually administered preoperatively for thyroid surgery as it decreases the vascularity of the gland.[46] Inorganic iodide should not be administered before thionamide treatment as it may initially increase the amount of thyroid hormone released and precipitate thyroid storm (Jod-Basedow effect). Anesthetic agents that are vagolytic or sympathomimetic (eg, pancuronium, ephedrine, epinephrine, norepinephrine, atropine) are best avoided in patients with thyrotoxicosis.[19]

The most feared perioperative complication that usually arises from either undiagnosed or undertreated hyperthyroidism is thyroid storm. Thyroid storm can occur any time in the perioperative period, although it usually occurs either intraoperatively or in the first 48 hours postoperatively. The mortality of thyroid storm is 10% to 75% and it requires monitoring in a critical-care environment.[47] Symptoms are nonspecific and include hyperpyrexia up to 41.1°C (106°F), tachycardia, and delirium.[48] Other conditions that should be considered on the differential diagnosis include malignant hyperthermia, neuroleptic malignant syndrome, and pheochromocytoma. As the mortality of this entity is high if left untreated and the diagnosis is purely clinical (supported by laboratory data), it is often necessary to treat empirically before confirmation.[49] Treatment of thyroid storm includes thionamides, β-blockers (goal heart rate <90 beats per minute), and antipyretics (or external cooling measures).[19] Acetaminophen is preferred to salicylates as the latter may exacerbate thyrotoxicosis by decreasing thyroid protein binding and increasing free T_3 and T_4.[49] A search for the precipitating cause of thyroid storm should be undertaken immediately. The most common cause in the perioperative period is infection (sepsis). Blood, urine, and sputum cultures should be obtained; however, empiric antibiotics are not recommended.[50] For those patients who are volume depleted, particularly if chronic hyperthyroidism exists, volume resuscitation with the addition of dextrose should be administered to replace depleted glycogen stores.[51]

HYPOTHYROIDISM

Hypothyroidism is a common endocrinopathy in the United States that affects about 1% of all patients and is more prevalent in females.[47] Primary hypothyroidism accounts for 95% of all cases and is characterized by low thyroid hormone levels (free T_4 <5 pmol/L) in the face of normal or increased TSH (often >10 mU/L). Common signs and symptoms of hypothyroidism include lethargy, fatigue, anorexia, headaches, hoarse voice, depression, and cold intolerance. The most common noniatrogenic cause is chronic autoimmune thyroiditis (Hashimoto thyroiditis). There are myriad iatrogenic causes with which the perioperative clinician needs to be familiar. Surgical thyroid resection or radioactive ablations are common causes that can frequently be anticipated. Less obvious, however, are treatment of hyperthyroidism or other pituitary and hypothalamic disorders (Sheehan syndrome, pituitary dysfunction after head trauma).[52] Various drugs can induce hypothyroidism, including lithium, amiodarone, iron, and cholestyramine. The surgical stress response in addition to general anesthesia may also incite hypothyroidism or, more commonly, the classis euthyroid sick syndrome.[53] After induction of general anesthesia, total T_3 levels decrease and remain low for at least 24 hours.[54] Understanding the implications of hypothyroidism on the morbidity and mortality of surgical patients may allow the perioperative clinician to anticipate complications and preemptively manage them.[55]

Similar to hyperthyroidism, hypothyroidism affects multiple organ systems and encompasses a wide clinical spectrum. The most clinically important of these is the cardiovascular system. Although plasma catecholamine levels are generally within normal limits, β-adrenergic receptor function is depressed and results in an imbalance of α- and β-adrenergic activity, with α predominating. In general, a deficiency in thyroid activity culminates in depressed cardiac function (inotropy and chronotropy), and increased systemic vascular resistance. The pulmonary system is affected as there may be depressed responses to hypercarbia and hypoxemia[56] and, in more severe cases, decreased lung diffusion capacity.[57] The renin-angiotensin-aldosterone complex responds to this situation by excreting sodium (> free water) culminating in hyponatremia and intravascular volume depletion.

The preferred treatment of hypothyroidism is tetraiodothyronine (T_4, levothyroxine) replacement and patients should preferably be rendered euthyroid before surgery. The more active hormone (T_3) is less stable but is converted in vivo intracellularly. The half-life of levothyroxine is approximately 1 week and therefore it is not imperative that patients take their dose the morning of surgery.[42] If intravenous dosing is necessary, half the enteral dose is equivalent. There is controversy in hypothyroid patients with known ischemic heart disease or presenting for coronary revascularization. Rapid replenishment of thyroid function risks increasing myocardial oxygen demand, causing ischemia. However, delay in therapy may place the patient at risk of developing myxedema coma.[58] Currently, the consensus is that if a patient needs urgent cardiac revascularization, they should undergo the procedure before replacement therapy[59,60]; however, many endocrinologists recommend starting at least low dose T_4 in consultation with the cardiologist.

Patients presenting for surgery with hypothyroidism can be grouped into 3 categories: (1) hypothyroid patients well controlled on thyroid medications, (2) mild to moderately hypothyroid patients, and (3) patients presenting with or developing severe hypothyroidism (myxedema coma) perioperatively. There is little to do with the first group other than be aware of their thyroid replacement dosing and be hyper-acute to signs and symptoms of worsening hypothyroidism postoperatively, including delirium, prolonged ileus, infection without fever, and myxedema coma. Preoperative sedation in this group should be minimized as these patients can be exquisitely sensitive to narcotics and benzodiazepines. Most patients with mild to moderate hypothyroidism can undergo surgery without a disproportionate increase in perioperative risk.[55,60,61] Close attention to airway patency in the postoperative period is necessary as there have been reports of airway obstruction in hypothyroid patients.[62] Intraoperative fluid replacement should be with dextrose containing normal saline. Controlled ventilation is recommended as these patients are at risk for hypoventilation. In those patients who present for surgery with severe hypothyroidism (depressed mental status, pericardial effusion, and heart failure) or in whom treatment is deemed necessary before urgent/emergent surgery (severely depressed T_4 and T_3), intravenous levothyroxine (200–500 μg given during 30 minutes) should be administered, followed by a daily dose of 50 to 100 μg intravenously.[63] As many patients with hypothyroidism also have adrenal insufficiency (and because thyroid replacement may precipitate adrenal crisis), glucocorticoids should be administered concurrently.[19]

Myxedema coma is rare and usually presents postoperatively. It is commonly precipitated by additional insults such as infection, cold exposure, sedatives, analgesics, and various other medications. Although the mortality of this entity has been reported to be as high as 80%, it seems to be decreasing in recent years likely because of increased awareness and improved diagnostic testing.[59,64,65] Myxedema coma is characterized by severely depressed mental status (sometimes coma or seizure), hypothermia, bradycardia, hyponatremia, heart failure, and hypopnea. Although maintenance of normothermia is tempting, the resulting vasodilatation may cause cardiovascular collapse in someone with intravascular volume depletion, cardiac insufficiency, and pericardial effusion/tamponade and should be performed extremely carefully, if at all.[59] Myxedema coma is a medical emergency and necessitates urgent administration of levothyroxine. An initial intravenous bolus of 200 to 500 μg should be given followed by 50 to 100 μg/d. Dehydration is frequently present and aggressive volume resuscitation with dextrose and normal saline should be instituted. Again, intravenous glucocorticoids should be administered (eg, 50 mg hydrocortisone 4 times a day) because of frequent concomitant adrenal insufficiency. Resolution of symptoms, if properly treated, should be seen within 24 hours.

ADRENAL INSUFFICIENCY

The hypothalamic-pituitary-adrenal (HPA) axis is central to a patient's ability to generate a surgical stress response. A defect anywhere in this cycle has dramatic consequences in the perioperative period. Whereas tuberculosis used to be the main cause of primary adrenal insufficiency (AI), autoimmune adrenalitis is now the most common cause. Other causes of primary AI include infections, adrenalectomy, and sepsis.[66,67] However, of greater importance to perioperative clinicians is secondary AI. Secondary AI is characterized by atrophy of the adrenal cortex and occurs when insufficient adrenocorticotrophic hormone (ACTH) is released to stimulate the adrenal cortex. It is most commonly caused by exogenous glucocorticoid administration, which suppresses hypothalamic corticotrophin-releasing hormone and pituitary ACTH. Although there is remarkable variability in individual response to a particular dose and length of treatment with steroids, in general any patient who has received the equivalent of 20 mg per day of prednisone for greater than 5 days is at risk for suppression of the HPA axis and if they have been on therapy for approximately 1 month they may have HPA suppression for up to 6 to 12 months after stopping therapy.[68–70] Likewise, an equivalent dose of prednisone 5 mg (or less) for any period of time will not usually suppress the HPA axis significantly.[71] Other modes of steroid administration should be noted preoperatively as topical, inhaled, and regional administration of glucocorticoids may all cause adrenal suppression.[72] In addition, these generalizations pertain to the patient taking steroids in the morning. A lower dose of steroids in the evening may inhibit the normal diurnal ACTH release and affect the way that patient is able to respond to a surgical stress.[72]

Although glucocorticoids alone are not vasoactive, they mediate vascular tone by increasing responsiveness to catecholamines. This effect occurs at a local tissue level (ie, not centrally mediated) and likely is mediated by inhibition of prostacyclin production.[73,74] Mineralocorticoid deficiency does not have the same effect. Mineralocorticoid (ie. aldosterone) secretion is primarily regulated by the renin-angiotensin system. A deficiency in ACTH (by glucocorticoid administration) will not result in aldosterone deficiency.[72]

Tests to detect perioperative adrenal suppression or identify patients who will respond to supplemental glucocorticoids have been neither sensitive nor specific.[72,75–77] However, the short ACTH stimulation test is able to assess adrenocortical function reliably.[75,78] If this test is abnormal preoperatively, supplemental perioperative glucocorticoid administration is justified. If the risk for perioperative adrenal suppression is significant a systematic approach should be taken to determine if steroid supplementation is necessary (**Fig. 3**). The decision should be based on suspicion (from history and physical examination), acuity of the operation, and anticipated severity of the procedure. If there is a high suspicion for the presence or development of AI and the procedure is emergent, steroids should be administered. If there is less urgency and time allows, an ACTH stimulation test should be performed to see if the adrenal gland appropriately responds to supraphysiologic doses of ACTH. Even if a preoperative ACTH stimulation test is normal and the patient is at high risk for perioperative AI, if unexplained hypotension persists despite volume repletion, steroids should be administered in a dose consistent with the level of injury. Postoperatively, steroids should be continued until the stress response diminishes (usually 48 hours).[79] The presence of unexplained nausea, vomiting, hypotension, orthostasis, change in mental status, hyponatremia, or hyperkalemia should warrant checking T_4, TSH, and random plasma cortisol and, depending on the urgency of the situation, may require empiric therapy with stress-dose steroids and possibly T_4. In addition, recrudescence of a stressor (eg, postoperative infection) may warrant reinstitution of supplemental glucocorticoids.

One drug that warrants mention in patients suspected of or at high risk of AI is etomidate. Etomidate is a frequently used anesthetic induction agent. Although it is a particularly attractive option for patients who are hemodynamically unstable, its effect of inhibiting steroid synthesis may precipitate acute AI and is best avoided in this population.[80,81]

PHEOCHROMOCYTOMA

Pheochromocytomas are rare neuroendocrine tumors, usually located in the adrenal medulla (although they may be found in extra-adrenal tissues) originating in catecholamine-producing chromaffin cells. The 10-10-10 rule is a reminder that 10% of these tumors are bilateral, 10% are extra-adrenal, and less than 10% are malignant. Most pheochromocytomas synthesize and secrete norepinephrine, although hypersecretion of epinephrine can also be seen. Signs and symptoms include periodic flushing, palpitations, sweating, headaches, and hypertension. Patients usually present

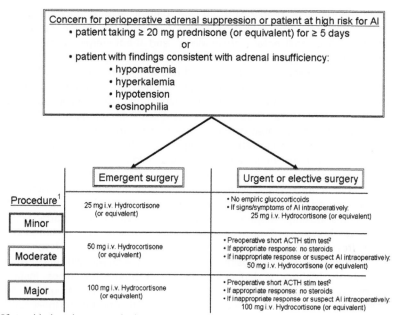

Concern for perioperative adrenal suppression or patient at high risk for AI
- patient taking ≥ 20 mg prednisone (or equivalent) for ≥ 5 days
  or
- patient with findings consistent with adrenal insufficiency:
  - hyponatremia
  - hyperkalemia
  - hypotension
  - eosinophilia

Procedure[1]	Emergent surgery	Urgent or elective surgery
Minor	25 mg i.v. Hydrocortisone (or equivalent)	• No empiric glucocorticoids • If signs/symptoms of AI intraoperatively: 25 mg i.v. Hydrocortisone (or equivalent)
Moderate	50 mg i.v. Hydrocortisone (or equivalent)	• Preoperative short ACTH stim test[2] • If appropriate response: no steroids • If inappropriate response or suspect AI intraoperatively: 50 mg i.v. Hydrocortisone (or equivalent)
Major	100 mg i.v. Hydrocortisone (or equivalent)	• Preoperative short ACTH stim test[2] • If appropriate response: no steroids • If inappropriate response or suspect AI intraoperatively: 100 mg i.v. Hydrocortisone (or equivalent)

* If steroid given intraoperatively:
--> Continue q 8 hour dosing for 48 hours
--> If continued need, consider endocrine consultation

Fig. 3. Algorithm for perioperative steroid administration. [1]Minor procedures include those performed under local anesthesia or those less than 1 hour in duration; moderate procedures include most vascular surgeries or orthopedic procedures; major procedures include larger prolonged operations such as esophagectomy or those using cardiopulmonary bypass. [2]The short ACTH stimulation involves administration of 250 μg i.v. synthetic ACTH (Cortrosyn, cosyntropin) followed by a plasma cortisol collection in 30 minutes. A plasma cortisol concentration greater than 18 to 20 μg/dL is consistent with normal adrenal function. i.v., intravenous; stim, stimulation. (*Adapted from* Kohl BA, Schwartz S. Surgery in the patient with endocrine dysfunction. Anesthesiol Clin 2009;27(4):687–703; with permission.)

perioperatively for (not despite) their pheochromocytoma. However, some patients may present with their first catecholamine crisis during routine surgery and thus familiarity with this syndrome is critical.

If a diagnosis of pheochromocytoma is suspected, the initial recommended test is measurement of plasma-free metanephrines, as the sensitivity is reportedly 99%.[82] Thus, a negative test essentially excludes this diagnosis. Urinary vanillylmandelic acid levels have much higher specificity (95%). Once there is biochemical evidence of a catecholamine-secreting tumor, radiographic imaging studies are performed to localize the tumor (usually magnetic resonance imaging or nuclear imaging).[83]

The end-organ that is most negatively affected in this syndrome is the cardiovascular system. Chronic, often severe, hypertension can frequently be corroborated with abnormal electrocardiography (ECG) findings (repolarization abnormalities, ventricular hypertrophy, nonspecific ST-T wave changes, and QTc interval prolongation). Some of these abnormalities will resolve after removal of the tumor.[84] The most common condition seen in these patients is a hypertrophic cardiomyopathy secondary to norepinephrine-induced hypertension. As most of these tumors are nonmalignant, surgery may be curative in more than 90% of cases.[85]

Careful preoperative preparation for the patient with pheochromocytoma is necessary. Failure to premedicate properly can increase perioperative mortality dramatically.[85] The goal entails adequate α- and β-adrenergic blockade. Current recommendations are that phenoxybenzamine (a long-acting noncompetitive α-adrenergic antagonist) be initiated approximately 1 to 2 weeks preoperatively.[86,87] Because the half-life of this drug is 24 to 36 hours, patients often require large amounts of intravenous fluid postoperatively and may be somnolent during this time because of central α_2-adrenoceptor blockade. Roizen and colleagues[88] recommended the following criteria for establishing adequate preoperative α-adrenergic blockade: (1) blood pressure should be no higher than 160/90 mmHg in the 24 hours preoperatively, (2) orthostatic hypotension should be present, (3) there should be no ST-T wave changes on ECG for 1 week preoperatively, and (4) there should be no more than 1 premature ventricular contraction every 5 minutes. For those patients with persistent tachycardia or hypertension, a β-blocker can be initiated 3 to 5 days before surgery.[59] There is a theoretic risk of inciting unopposed α-agonism if β-antagonists are started first, culminating in severely increased vascular resistance. Metyrosine (a competitive inhibitor of tyrosine hydroxylase) has also been used successfully preoperatively. Tyrosine hydroxylase facilitates conversion of tyrosine to Dopa, and is the rate-limiting step in catecholamine synthesis. Metyrosine depletes tumor stores of catecholamines. Institution of early α-antagonism in addition to realization that these patients are frequently severely hypovolemic has dramatically decreased the perioperative mortality in these patients.[89] Echocardiography can be valuable in detecting overall systolic and diastolic function. Left ventricular hypertrophy is present in most of these patients; however, ventricular dilatation is a more ominous sign. For this reason, some have suggested obtaining a preoperative echocardiogram regardless of blood pressure.[90]

Attempts to minimize hemodynamic fluctuations pre- and intraoperatively are advisable. Sufficient preoperative anxiolysis is warranted. In addition to standard monitors, careful hemodynamic monitoring is necessary and an intra-arterial catheter should be placed before anesthetic induction. Furthermore, several large-bore intravenous catheters should be placed (rapid volume administration is often necessary) and serious consideration should be given to central intravenous access for administration of vasoactive medications.[91] Placement of a pulmonary artery catheter is not necessary, although may be helpful in the presence of significant cardiac disease.[92,93] Agents that either directly or indirectly increase catecholamine levels, such as ketamine and ephedrine, should be avoided. In addition, morphine (which causes histamine release) has been associated with and felt to be a trigger of pheochromocytoma crisis.[94] Meperidine and droperidol have also been associated with severe hypertension and are best avoided.[95] Intraoperative hypertensive crises are best treated with rapid-acting direct vasodilators (eg, nitroprusside, nitroglycerine, nicardipine).

Postoperatively these patients may continue to be hypertensive for up to 1 week because of increased catecholamine levels in adrenergic nerve endings. Alternatively, aggressive preoperative adrenergic blockade may render the patient hypotensive postoperatively, usually for 24 to 48 hours, at which point most of the phenoxybenzamine has been eliminated. An improved understanding of the pathophysiology of this disease in addition to numerous investigations studying various techniques has dramatically improved perioperative outcome.[86]

SUMMARY

Patients with endocrine dysfunction present unique challenges to perioperative clinicians. DM is the most common endocrinopathy in patients presenting for surgery.

Numerous investigations have shown that the increased mortality formerly seen in these patients can be dramatically minimized (compared with their counterparts without DM) with careful glycemic management. It is always advisable to normalize, as best as possible, the endocrinopathy or hemodynamic consequences before surgery (particularly in hypo- and hyperthyroidism, and pheochromocytoma). AI often presents intra- or postoperatively and thus being familiar with the signs and symptoms allows the perioperative clinician to be acutely aware and institute immediate therapy if necessary.

REFERENCES

1. Glister BC, Vigersky RA. Perioperative management of type 1 diabetes mellitus. Endocrinol Metab Clin North Am 2003;32:411–36.
2. Gavin LA. Perioperative management of the diabetic patient. Endocrinol Metab Clin North Am 1992;21:457–75.
3. Umpierrez GE, Isaacs SD, Bazargan N, et al. Hyperglycemia: an independent marker of in-hospital mortality in patients with undiagnosed diabetes. J Clin Endocrinol Metab 2002;87:978–82.
4. Kim KS, Kim SK, Lee YK, et al. Diagnostic value of glycated haemoglobin for the early detection of diabetes in high-risk subjects. Diabet Med 2008;25:997–1000.
5. Furnary AP, Zerr KJ, Grunkemeier GL, et al. Continuous intravenous insulin infusion reduces the incidence of deep sternal wound infection in diabetic patients after cardiac surgical procedures. Ann Thorac Surg 1999;67:352–60 [discussion: 60–2].
6. Zerr KJ, Furnary AP, Grunkemeier GL, et al. Glucose control lowers the risk of wound infection in diabetics after open heart operations. Ann Thorac Surg 1997;63:356–61.
7. Pozzilli P, Leslie RD. Infections and diabetes: mechanisms and prospects for prevention. Diabet Med 1994;11:935–41.
8. Latham R, Lancaster AD, Covington JF, et al. The association of diabetes and glucose control with surgical-site infections among cardiothoracic surgery patients. Infect Control Hosp Epidemiol 2001;22:607–12.
9. Nathan DM, Singer DE, Hurxthal K, et al. The clinical information value of the glycosylated hemoglobin assay. N Engl J Med 1984;310:341–6.
10. Stevens LA, Coresh J, Greene T, et al. Assessing kidney function–measured and estimated glomerular filtration rate. N Engl J Med 2006;354:2473–83.
11. Reissell E, Orko R, Maunuksela EL, et al. Predictability of difficult laryngoscopy in patients with long-term diabetes mellitus. Anaesthesia 1990;45:1024–7.
12. Hogan K, Rusy D, Springman SR. Difficult laryngoscopy and diabetes mellitus. Anesth Analg 1988;67:1162–5.
13. Monk TG, Mueller M, White PF. Treatment of stress response during balanced anesthesia. Comparative effects of isoflurane, alfentanil, and trimethaphan. Anesthesiology 1992;76:39–45.
14. American Diabetes Association. Standards of medical care in diabetes–2007. Diabetes Care 2007;30(Suppl 1):S4–41.
15. American Association of Clinical Endocrinologists medical guidelines for clinical practice for the management of diabetes mellitus. Available at: http://www.aace. com/pub/pdf/guidelines/DMGuidelines2007.pdf. Accessed November 9, 2009.
16. Garber AJ, Moghissi ES, Bransome ED Jr, et al. American College of Endocrinology position statement on inpatient diabetes and metabolic control. Endocr Pract 2004;10(Suppl 2):4–9.

17. Kosiborod M, Inzucchi SE, Krumholz HM, et al. Glucometrics in patients hospitalized with acute myocardial infarction: defining the optimal outcomes-based measure of risk. Circulation 2008;117:1018–27.
18. Pinto DS, Skolnick AH, Kirtane AJ, et al. U-shaped relationship of blood glucose with adverse outcomes among patients with ST-segment elevation myocardial infarction. J Am Coll Cardiol 2005;46:178–80.
19. Mercado DL, Petty BG. Perioperative medication management. Med Clin North Am 2003;87:41–57.
20. Metchick LN, Petit WA Jr, Inzucchi SE. Inpatient management of diabetes mellitus. Am J Med 2002;113:317–23.
21. Marks JB. Perioperative management of diabetes. Am Fam Physician 2003;67: 93–100.
22. Lambillotte C, Gilon P, Henquin JC. Direct glucocorticoid inhibition of insulin secretion. An in vitro study of dexamethasone effects in mouse islets. J Clin Invest 1997;99:414–23.
23. Chia CW, Egan JM. Special features: incretin-based therapies in type 2 diabetes mellitus. J Clin Endocrinol Metab 2008;93(10):3703–16.
24. Gautier JF, Choukem SP, Girard J. Physiology of incretins (GIP and GLP-1) and abnormalities in type 2 diabetes. Diabetes Metab 2008;34(Suppl 2): S65–72.
25. Doenst T, Wijeysundera D, Karkouti K, et al. Hyperglycemia during cardiopulmonary bypass is an independent risk factor for mortality in patients undergoing cardiac surgery. J Thorac Cardiovasc Surg 2005;130:1144.
26. Gandhi GY, Nuttall GA, Abel MD, et al. Intensive intraoperative insulin therapy versus conventional glucose management during cardiac surgery: a randomized trial. Ann Intern Med 2007;146:233–43.
27. Gandhi GY, Nuttall GA, Abel MD, et al. Intraoperative hyperglycemia and perioperative outcomes in cardiac surgery patients. Mayo Clin Proc 2005;80: 862–6.
28. Lazar HL, Chipkin SR, Fitzgerald CA, et al. Tight glycemic control in diabetic coronary artery bypass graft patients improves perioperative outcomes and decreases recurrent ischemic events. Circulation 2004;109:1497–502.
29. Ouattara A, Lecomte P, Le Manach Y, et al. Poor intraoperative blood glucose control is associated with a worsened hospital outcome after cardiac surgery in diabetic patients. Anesthesiology 2005;103:687–94.
30. Puskas F, Grocott HP, White WD, et al. Intraoperative hyperglycemia and cognitive decline after CABG. Ann Thorac Surg 2007;84:1467–73.
31. Fleisher LA, Beckman JA, Brown KA, et al. ACC/AHA 2007 guidelines on perioperative cardiovascular evaluation and care for noncardiac surgery: a report of the American College of Cardiology/American Heart Association Task Force on Practice Guidelines (Writing Committee to Revise the 2002 Guidelines on Perioperative Cardiovascular Evaluation for Noncardiac Surgery): developed in collaboration with the American Society of Echocardiography, American Society of Nuclear Cardiology, Heart Rhythm Society, Society of Cardiovascular Anesthesiologists, Society for Cardiovascular Angiography and Interventions, Society for Vascular Medicine and Biology, and Society for Vascular Surgery. Circulation 2007;116:e418–99.
32. Swift CS, Boucher JL. Nutrition therapy for the hospitalized patient with diabetes. Endocr Pract 2006;12(Suppl 3):61–7.
33. van den Berghe G, Wouters P, Weekers F, et al. Intensive insulin therapy in the critically ill patients. N Engl J Med 2001;345:1359–67.

34. Golden SH, Peart-Vigilance C, Kao WH, et al. Perioperative glycemic control and the risk of infectious complications in a cohort of adults with diabetes. Diabetes Care 1999;22:1408–14.

35. Treggiari MM, Karir V, Yanez ND, et al. Intensive insulin therapy and mortality in critically ill patients. Crit Care 2008;12:R29.

36. De La Rosa GD, Donado JH, Restrepo AH, et al. Strict glycemic control in patients hospitalized in a mixed medical and surgical intensive care unit: a randomized clinical trial. Crit Care 2008;12:R120.

37. Klein I, Danzi S. Thyroid disease and the heart. Circulation 2007;116: 1725–35.

38. Biondi B, Palmieri EA, Lombardi G, et al. Effects of thyroid hormone on cardiac function: the relative importance of heart rate, loading conditions, and myocardial contractility in the regulation of cardiac performance in human hyperthyroidism. J Clin Endocrinol Metab 2002;87:968–74.

39. Forfar JC, Muir AL, Sawers SA, et al. Abnormal left ventricular function in hyperthyroidism: evidence for a possible reversible cardiomyopathy. N Engl J Med 1982;307:1165–70.

40. Woeber KA. Thyrotoxicosis and the heart. N Engl J Med 1992;327:94–8.

41. Klein I, Ojamaa K. Thyroid hormone and the cardiovascular system. N Engl J Med 2001;344:501–9.

42. Spell NO 3rd. Stopping and restarting medications in the perioperative period. Med Clin North Am 2001;85:1117–28.

43. Furlong D, Ahmed I, Jabbour S. Perioperative management of endocrine disorders. In: Merli GJ, Weitz HH, editors. Medical management of the surgical patient. 3rd edition. Philadelphia: Elsevier Saunders; 2007. Chapter 12.

44. Farwell AP, Braverman LE. Thyroid and antithyroid drugs. In: Hardman JG, Limberd LE, editors. Goodman and Gilman's: the pharmacological basis of therapeutics. 10th edition. New York: McGraw-Hill; 2001. p. 1563–96.

45. Markou K, Georgopoulos N, Kyriazopoulou V, et al. Iodine-induced hypothyroidism. Thyroid 2001;11:501–10.

46. Streetman DD, Khanderia U. Diagnosis and treatment of Graves disease. Ann Pharmacother 2003;37:1100–9.

47. Ringel MD. Management of hypothyroidism and hyperthyroidism in the intensive care unit. Crit Care Clin 2001;17:59–74.

48. Howton JC. Thyroid storm presenting as coma. Ann Emerg Med 1988;17:343–5.

49. McKeown NJ, Tews MC, Gossain VV, et al. Hyperthyroidism. Emerg Med Clin North Am 2005;23:669–85, viii.

50. Burch HB, Wartofsky L. Life-threatening thyrotoxicosis. Thyroid storm. Endocrinol Metab Clin North Am 1993;22:263–77.

51. Nayak B, Burman K. Thyrotoxicosis and thyroid storm. Endocrinol Metab Clin North Am 2006;35:663–86, vii.

52. Benvenga S, Campenni A, Ruggeri RM, et al. Clinical review 113: hypopituitarism secondary to head trauma. J Clin Endocrinol Metab 2000;85:1353–61.

53. Wellby ML, Kennedy JA, Barreau PB, et al. Endocrine and cytokine changes during elective surgery. J Clin Pathol 1994;47:1049–51.

54. Stathatos N, Wartofsky L. Perioperative management of patients with hypothyroidism. Endocrinol Metab Clin North Am 2003;32:503–18.

55. Ladenson PW, Levin AA, Ridgway EC, et al. Complications of surgery in hypothyroid patients. Am J Med 1984;77:261–6.

56. Zwillich CW, Pierson DJ, Hofeldt FD, et al. Ventilatory control in myxedema and hypothyroidism. N Engl J Med 1975;292:662–5.

57. Wilson WR, Bedell GN. The pulmonary abnormalities in myxedema. J Clin Invest 1960;39:42–55.
58. O'Connor CJ, March R, Tuman KJ. Severe myxedema after cardiopulmonary bypass. Anesth Analg 2003;96:62–4.
59. Connery LE, Coursin DB. Assessment and therapy of selected endocrine disorders. Anesthesiol Clin North America 2004;22:93–123.
60. Schiff RL, Welsh GA. Perioperative evaluation and management of the patient with endocrine dysfunction. Med Clin North Am 2003;87:175–92.
61. Weinberg AD, Brennan MD, Gorman CA, et al. Outcome of anesthesia and surgery in hypothyroid patients. Arch Intern Med 1983;143:893–7.
62. Benfari G, de Vincentiis M. Postoperative airway obstruction: a complication of a previously undiagnosed hypothyroidism. Otolaryngol Head Neck Surg 2005; 132:343–4.
63. Bennett-Guerrero E, Kramer DC, Schwinn DA. Effect of chronic and acute thyroid hormone reduction on perioperative outcome. Anesth Analg 1997;85:30–6.
64. Wartofsky L. Myxedema coma. Endocrinol Metab Clin North Am 2006;35:687–98, vii–viii.
65. Dutta P, Bhansali A, Masoodi SR, et al. Predictors of outcome in myxoedema coma: a study from a tertiary care centre. Crit Care 2008;12:R1.
66. Arlt W, Allolio B. Adrenal insufficiency. Lancet 2003;361:1881–93.
67. Shenker Y, Skatrud JB. Adrenal insufficiency in critically ill patients. Am J Respir Crit Care Med 2001;163:1520–3.
68. Nicholson G, Burrin JM, Hall GM. Peri-operative steroid supplementation. Anaesthesia 1998;53:1091–104.
69. Henzen C, Suter A, Lerch E, et al. Suppression and recovery of adrenal response after short-term, high-dose glucocorticoid treatment. Lancet 2000;355:542–5.
70. Hopkins RL, Leinung MC. Exogenous Cushing's syndrome and glucocorticoid withdrawal. Endocrinol Metab Clin North Am 2005;34:371–84, ix.
71. Jabbour SA. Steroids and the surgical patient. Med Clin North Am 2001;85: 1311–7.
72. Axelrod L. Perioperative management of patients treated with glucocorticoids. Endocrinol Metab Clin North Am 2003;32:367–83.
73. Axelrod L. Inhibition of prostacyclin production mediates permissive effect of glucocorticoids on vascular tone. Perturbations of this mechanism contribute to pathogenesis of Cushing's syndrome and Addison's disease. Lancet 1983;1: 904–6.
74. Rascher W, Dietz R, Schomig A, et al. Reversal of corticosterone-induced supersensitivity of vascular smooth muscle to noradrenaline by arachidonic acid and prostacyclin. Eur J Pharmacol 1980;68:267–73.
75. Kehlet H, Binder C. Value of an ACTH test in assessing hypothalamic-pituitary-adrenocortical function in glucocorticoid-treated patients. Br Med J 1973;2:147–9.
76. Knudsen L, Christiansen LA, Lorentzen JE. Hypotension during and after operation in glucocorticoid-treated patients. Br J Anaesth 1981;53:295–301.
77. Plumpton FS, Besser GM, Cole PV. Corticosteroid treatment and surgery. 1. An investigation of the indications for steroid cover. Anaesthesia 1969;24:3–11.
78. Lindholm J, Kehlet H. Re-evaluation of the clinical value of the 30 min ACTH test in assessing the hypothalamic-pituitary-adrenocortical function. Clin Endocrinol (Oxf) 1987;26:53–9.
79. Salem M, Tainsh RE Jr, Bromberg J, et al. Perioperative glucocorticoid coverage. A reassessment 42 years after emergence of a problem. Ann Surg 1994;219: 416–25.

80. Thomas Z, Fraser GL. An update on the diagnosis of adrenal insufficiency and the use of corticotherapy in critical illness. Ann Pharmacother 2007;41:1456–65.
81. Wagner RL, White PF, Kan PB, et al. Inhibition of adrenal steroidogenesis by the anesthetic etomidate. N Engl J Med 1984;310:1415–21.
82. Lenders JW, Pacak K, Walther MM, et al. Biochemical diagnosis of pheochromocytoma: which test is best? JAMA 2002;287:1427–34.
83. Pacak K, Linehan WM, Eisenhofer G, et al. Recent advances in genetics, diagnosis, localization, and treatment of pheochromocytoma. Ann Intern Med 2001; 134:315–29.
84. Liao WB, Liu CF, Chiang CW, et al. Cardiovascular manifestations of pheochromocytoma. Am J Emerg Med 2000;18:622–5.
85. Plouin PF, Duclos JM, Soppelsa F, et al. Factors associated with perioperative morbidity and mortality in patients with pheochromocytoma: analysis of 165 operations at a single center. J Clin Endocrinol Metab 2001;86:1480–6.
86. Bravo EL. Pheochromocytoma. Curr Ther Endocrinol Metab 1997;6:195–7.
87. Newell KA, Prinz RA, Brooks MH, et al. Plasma catecholamine changes during excision of pheochromocytoma. Surgery 1988;104:1064–73.
88. Roizen MF, Schreider BD, Hassan SZ. Anesthesia for patients with pheochromocytoma. Anesthesiol Clin North America 1987;5:269–75.
89. Geoghegan JG, Emberton M, Bloom SR, et al. Changing trends in the management of phaeochromocytoma. Br J Surg 1998;85:117–20.
90. Bravo EL. Evolving concepts in the pathophysiology, diagnosis, and treatment of pheochromocytoma. Endocr Rev 1994;15:356–68.
91. Kinney MA, Warner ME, vanHeerden JA, et al. Perianesthetic risks and outcomes of pheochromocytoma and paraganglioma resection. Anesth Analg 2000;91: 1118–23.
92. Prys-Roberts C. Phaeochromocytoma–recent progress in its management. Br J Anaesth 2000;85:44–57.
93. Young JB, Landsberg L. Catecholamines and the adrenal medulla. In: Wilson JD, Foster DW, Kronenberg HM, et al, editors. Williams textbook of endocrinology. Philadelphia: Saunders; 1998. p. 705–28.
94. Jovenich JJ. Anesthesia in adrenal surgery. Urol Clin North Am 1989;16:583–7.
95. Kinney MA, Narr BJ, Warner MA. Perioperative management of pheochromocytoma. J Cardiothorac Vasc Anesth 2002;16:359–69.

Anesthesia for the Patient with Tracheal Stenosis

Geraldine Daumerie, MD[a], Stacey Su, MD[b],
E. Andrew Ochroch, MD, MSCE[a,b],*

KEYWORDS

• Tracheal stenosis • Anesthesia • Trauma • Intubation

The larynx ends at the inferior edge of the cricoid cartilage. The cervical trachea starts below the inferior border of the cricoid and extends to the sternal notch, and the thoracic trachea is located from the sternal notch down to the carina. In total, the trachea is composed of 18 to 22 cartilaginous rings, each being 0.5 cm wide in the adult. The trachea is approximately 12 cm long in men and 10 cm long in women. Normal diameter is about 1.8 to 2.5 cm. With hyperextension, up to 50% of the trachea can be above the sternal notch. Blood supply to the trachea is from the inferior thyroid, the internal thoracic, the supreme intercostal, and the bronchial arteries.

Stenosis of the trachea signifies a functional impairment, with peak expiratory flow rates changing from 100% in a normal trachea with a diameter of 2 cm to 30% in a trachea with a diameter of 5 mm.[1] Tracheal stenosis has multiple causes. Pediatric tracheal stenosis can be divided into acquired versus congenital forms. Acquired forms of pediatric tracheal stenosis include trauma, mostly related to endotracheal intubation or from tracheostomy-induced formation of granulation tissue. Up to 8% of the neonates who undergo prolonged intubation can go on to develop tracheal stenosis. Congenital forms of tracheal stenosis are classified by Cantrell and Guild[2] as generalized hypoplasia, funnel-like stenosis, and segmental stenosis. They can also be categorized based on the length of the stenotic segment and associated anomalies.[3] Congenital tracheal stenoses include tracheal webs, tracheal agenesis/atresia, tracheomalacia, and vascular malformations that extrinsically compress the trachea.[2,3]

[a] Department of Anesthesiology, Hospital of the University of Pennsylvania, University of Pennsylvania, 680 Dulles Building, 3400 Spruce Street, Philadelphia, PA 19104, USA
[b] Department of Surgery, Division of Thoracic Surgery, University of Pennsylvania, 3400 Spruce Street, Philadelphia, PA 19104, USA
* Corresponding author. Department of Anesthesiology, Hospital of the University of Pennsylvania, University of Pennsylvania, 680 Dulles Building, 3400 Spruce Street, Philadelphia, PA 19104.
E-mail address: ochrocha@uphs.upenn.edu

Anesthesiology Clin 28 (2010) 157–174
doi:10.1016/j.anclin.2010.01.010
1932-2275/10/$ – see front matter © 2010 Elsevier Inc. All rights reserved.

anesthesiology.theclinics.com

In adults, tracheal stenosis may result from trauma, benign or malignant neoplastic conditions, chronic inflammatory diseases (such as sarcoid and amyloid), collagen vascular diseases (such as Wegener granulomatosis), or external compression from mediastinal masses.[4] Also possible is idiopathic laryngotracheal stenosis, a rare disease, which occurs almost exclusively in women with no identifiable cause of airway stenosis.[5] The most common cause of tracheal stenosis, however, continues to be trauma from prolonged endotracheal intubation.[6] This sequela was first recognized during the poliomyelitis epidemic in the 1950s when prolonged mechanical ventilation was used.[7]

Cooper and Grillo[8,9] first studied tracheal stenosis at the cuff site and showed that the main cause was the pressure exerted by the cuff. Cuff pressures greater than 30 mm Hg cause mucosal ischemia by exceeding mucosal capillary perfusion. This area of ischemia can develop chondritis and granulation tissue, then heal by fibrosis, leading to progressive tracheal stenosis. Cuff-related strictures assume an eccentric circumferential configuration, in contrast to tracheostomy-related strictures, which have a V shape on account of the loss of the anterior cartilaginous arch. The incidence of tracheal damage can be reduced with the use of high-volume, low-pressure cuffs that minimize the pressure exerted on the trachea via a larger area of contact. However, despite the use of these cuffs, up to 11% of patients may still develop some degree of tracheal stenosis as shown in a prospective study of 150 critically ill patients.[10] As compared with tracheal stenosis, glottic stenosis as a result of intubation is usually present posteriorly and can be associated with arytenoid cartilage dislocation, vocal cord paralysis, and granulomas. Bogdasarian and Olson[11] have classified this type of glottic stenosis based on location and involvement of vocal cords.

Another way of categorizing tracheal stenosis is on the basis of spectrum of fixed to dynamic collapse.[3] A fixed stenosis is typically a fibrotic segment of the trachea. As discussed in the "Physics of airflow" section, the Bernoulli principle holds that as air accelerates through a small orifice, the pressure will drop. Because the membranous surface of the trachea is flexible and mobile, it can be drawn up into the trachea. When this occurs, the actual airway compromise is greater than that which is simply predicted by the stenotic opening. Dynamic collapse from a prolapsing membranous wall can produce tracheal stenosis in patients without any fixed tracheal narrowing. These patients often have increased work of breathing as a result of chronic obstructive pulmonary disease (COPD), reactive airways disease, and/or obesity. Airway collapse can be on inspiration because of the pressure drop of airflow or on expiration because of the increased velocity of the airflow and the increased abdominal pressure, causing herniation of the membranous wall into the airway.

Tracheomalacia, literally "softening of the trachea," is a condition in which there has been a weakening of the cartilaginous structures of the trachea.[12,13] Typical causes are rheumatic (polychondritis), infectious, secondary to external beam radiation, and secondary to trauma or surgery.[12] There can be stenosis from partial collapse. Airflow can be limited on inspiration and on forced expiration, the latter being due to increased velocity of the airflow and increased abdominal pressure, causing prolapse of the membranous wall into the airway.

PHYSICS OF AIRFLOW
Principles of Flow

Flow through a tube, whether through the trachea, circulation, or any other orifice, can be difficult to measure. It is important to distinguish between flow and velocity, which are often confused. Flow, often denoted as Q, is defined as the volume passing a particular surface area per unit of time and is often denoted as mL/s or L/min, whereas velocity is the speed of fluid at a particular point in space. Flowing fluids in tubes possess velocity and pressure that can be used to analyze incompressible flow by using the Bernoulli equation, which states that

$$P + \frac{1}{2}\rho U^2 = P_0$$

where P is pressure, ρ is fluid density, U is velocity, and P_0 is a constant pressure. In this form of the Bernoulli equation, pressure decreases as velocity increases. In the flow inside a tube, velocity decreases as area increases.

Flow can be measured using the average velocity of the fluid across a tube. In laminar flow, the velocity has a parabolic shape, with slower velocities along the edges because of friction (**Fig. 1**), whereas turbulent flow has a flattened velocity profile. Turbulent flow is inefficient, and the energy needed to move a given volume is greater for turbulent flow than for laminar flow.

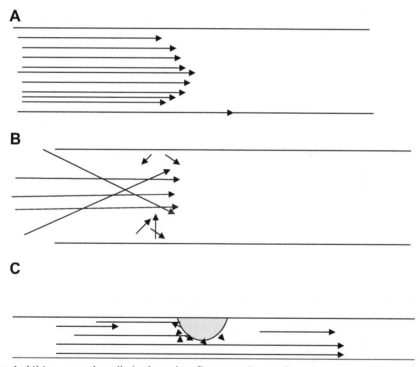

Fig. 1. (*A*) In a smooth-walled tube at low flow rates (ie, small pressure gradients), the flow rate is laminar; that is, flow moves smoothly in concentric circles, with the centermost area having the greatest flow velocity and the area nearest the wall of the tube being virtually stationary. (*B*) As the flow rate (and pressure gradient) increases, the flow transitions from laminar to turbulent. Instead of a neatly ordered flow, the velocities are more randomly distributed, and the energy needed for a given flow rate increases. Many factors govern this transition, including size of the tube, viscosity of the fluid, flow rate, and pressure gradient. These factors are combined in the determination of the Reynolds number. (*C*) Even at low flow rates, the distortion of laminar flow around an obstruction necessitates an increase in the pressure gradient to drive volumes greater than that simply predicted by the decrease in diameter. This is as a result of the effect of turbulent flow.

Most commonly, the flow that needs to be measured by anesthesiologists is not laminar, and the Bernoulli equation cannot be applied because it describes frictionless flows. The transition from laminar to turbulent flow depends on the type of fluid, the speed of the flow, and the shape of the flow. These fluid factors are combined in a ratio called the Reynolds number (Re).

$$Re = \rho UL/\mu$$

where ρ is the density of the fluid, U is the mean flow velocity, L is the characteristic length of the flow, and μ is the viscosity of the fluid. For flow through a tube of circular cross section, transition from laminar to turbulent flow occurs at a critical value of Re. A large Reynolds number indicates that viscous forces are not important at large scales of the flow. Using the definition of the Reynolds number, we can see that a large diameter with rapid flow, where the density of the fluid is high, tends toward turbulence. Also, rapid changes in diameter, as occurs in tracheal stenosis, may lead to turbulent flow. If flow in a tube passes through a sudden restriction, the turbulent flow is proportional to the area of the orifice and the square root of the pressure drop through the orifice as opposed to its direct proportionality to pressure gradient in laminar flow. Understanding the physics of airflow becomes an important concept in the diagnosis and treatment of tracheal stenosis.[14]

DIAGNOSIS OF TRACHEAL STENOSIS AND PREOPERATIVE EVALUATION
History and Physical Examination

As previously stated, tracheal stenosis can have numerous causes, with iatrogenic trauma being the most frequent cause. Other conditions that are related to tracheal stenosis should be ruled out. These include amyloidosis, Wegener granulomatosis, sarcoidosis, tuberculosis, and other infectious disease processes.[13] Patients can be tested for antinuclear cytoplasmic antigen to rule out Wegener granulomatosis. Rheumatology is often helpful in interpreting results and evaluating a patient for other collagen vascular diseases. A detailed history of the patient should be obtained, and a review of systems including difficulty clearing secretions, exercise tolerance, and orthopnea should be elicited. Physical examination should include palpation of the trachea, auscultation of the lungs and trachea, and evaluation of neck mobility. Routine blood work is all that is needed. Cardiac screening, such as an echocardiography or stress test, may be needed if the patient has had a change in symptoms or if the stenosis has rendered the patient incapable of activity.

A clear history of any antecedent airway management needs to be collected. A history of traumatic airway management can be surmised from prolonged hoarseness after an operation or from intubation in an emergent situation. All cases of postoperative or intensive care unit ventilation need to be examined for duration and the presence of other comorbidities, such as sepsis and heart failure, that have been associated with the development of tracheal stenosis.

Tracheal stenosis often presents with inspiratory stridor and/or expiratory wheezing. These patients are frequently misdiagnosed with asthma on initial presentation. These patients will be unresponsive to bronchodilators. Also, most patients with tracheal stenosis do not develop symptoms at rest until they have reached 70% stenosis.[15] On physical examination, patients may use accessory muscles or demonstrate tachypnea.

Flow-Volume Loops

Flow-volume loops can be useful in evaluating these patients. The flow-volume loops may show several anomalies: a delay in reaching peak expiratory flow, a truncation of peak expiratory and peak inspiratory flow, and/or an abrupt drop of expiratory flow at the end of expiration. In a patient with asthma, one can see flattening of the expiratory curve. This occurs predominantly late in expiration, with slowing of terminal flow rates. Peak flows are maintained, but the flow-volume curve becomes more convex toward the horizontal axis.[16]

On a flow-volume loop in a patient with a fixed upper airway obstruction such as tracheal stenosis, there is flattening of the inspiratory and the expiratory phases. The primary effect occurs early in expiration and results in a truncated, flat-topped flow-volume curve, with a normal late expiratory portion of the flow-volume curve.[17,18] It is important to remember that the quality of the flow-volume loops is totally dependent on the patient's effort and cooperation and that tracings obtained may not have the shapes presented earlier.[19]

Imaging

Imaging can be very useful in evaluating these patients. Chest radiographs can seem normal. Sometimes, a circumferential lesion can be seen on plain radiographs. Computed tomography (CT) scans can be an extremely useful diagnostic tool in these patients. However, it is important to obtain an airway CT rather than a neck or chest CT. A CT dedicated to the airways will evaluate the entire airway with thinner cuts. If thicker cuts are used, one can underestimate or miss the area of stenosis. Advances in imaging allow for 3-dimensional (3D) reconstruction of the trachea.[20] Multidetector CT is the imaging modality of choice. Multiplanar reformations and 3D images allow surgeons and interventional pulmonologists to select the adequate procedure for the patient. In tracheal stenosis secondary to prolonged intubation, one will see eccentric or concentric thickening, with associated luminal narrowing. Volume rendering techniques provide information on the length of stenosis and patency of the airways.[4] One may see a characteristic "hourglass" shape. In stenosis secondary to other causes, other findings consistent with the disease process can be evident on the CT scan: enlarged lymph nodes in fibrotic tuberculosis, thickening and calcification of tracheal rings in Wegener granulomatosis, and bronchial wall thickening in tracheobronchial amyloidosis. CT scans may demonstrate specific findings that can help narrow the differential diagnosis.

Endoscopy

Bronchoscopy remains the primary procedure in the diagnostic workup of tracheal stenosis and is the key in defining the characteristic features, extent, and location of the stenosis. Bronchoscopy in a patient with postintubation stenosis shows (1) circumferential luminal narrowing less than 2 cm in length, (2) a thin membrane that extends into the lumen, or (3) a long segment of eccentric soft tissue thickening.[12,21] Patients with stenosis related to tuberculosis will have granulation tissue with friable and ulcerated mucosa, whereas those with sarcoidosis may demonstrate a raised, cobblestoned appearance of the mucosa. Patients with Wegener granulomatosis may have inflammatory ulcers, plaques, or granulomatous tissues. Bronchoscopic findings in patients with amyloid may reveal thickened tracheal segments corresponding to areas of amyloid deposits. Patients may also have generalized mucosal edema and erythema on bronchoscopy.[22] Performing a fiberoptic bronchoscopy in an awake patient allows the physician to examine vocal cord function to determine if recurrent laryngeal nerve damage is present; it also allows for the evaluation of dynamic airway collapse with respiration. Bronchoscopic findings are not pathognomonic, and biopsies are often required to include or exclude an inflammatory disease process.

MANAGEMENT

The use of endoscopic treatment for the initial management of tracheal stenosis started in the 1980s, and bronchoscopic examination is paramount in patients with tracheal pathology. This examination will define the nature of the lesion, length, location, and degree of obstruction. If the obstruction is moderate to severe, bronchoscopic evaluation may be deferred until definitive treatment is chosen.[23] Rigid bronchoscopy is usually chosen in the nonsurgical treatment of these patients. Rigid bronchoscopy allows coring out of tumors, provides a means for ventilation, and may tamponade a source of bleeding.

Irradiation

Squamous cell carcinoma and adenoid cystic carcinoma respond to radiation. However, used alone, it is not a definitive treatment, and most tumors recur after a few years. However, radiation can be used as an adjunct to other methods.[24]

Dilatation

Dilatation can be used for the management of tracheal obstruction in emergency situations or in a planned approach to determine if surgical resection will be needed. Simple dilatation is often not a definite treatment as recurrence occurs. It should be used as a temporizing measure until more definitive treatment can be undertaken. Dilation is not recommended for mature, firm stenosis or those with cartilaginous components.[23] Ideally, it is performed under direct visualization and with a means of securing the airway. Dilatation can be performed with smooth round dilators, gradual dilation with ventilating bronchoscopes of increasing diameter, rigid bronchoscopes of increasing diameters, or dilating balloons passed through flexible bronchoscopes.[15,24] The risk of edema and mucosal trauma increases with multiple dilations, making this method of treatment less popular. Steroids can be used to minimize edema after these dilatations. Steroids can delay the synthesis of collagen in the early stages of scar formation. However, they can also delay wound healing and cause cartilage resorption.[23] In addition, local injection of steroids or mitomycin C may staunch the recurrence of scar formation at the site of stricture.

Laser

Lasers deliver energy to achieve cutting, coagulation, and vaporization with great precision and microhemostasis. The end result is less perioperative edema. The CO_2 laser has a wavelength of 10.6 μm and is used for lesions involving soft tissues. It can deliver power from less than 1 W to 100 W. When operating on the airways, it is used in the range of 3 to 6 W. However, the CO_2 laser cannot coagulate vessels larger than 0.5 mm in size and depends on an optic delivery system. Endoscopic laser treatment includes radial incision and dilation and excision.[21] Radial cuts are made into the fibrotic segment. This allows a planned tear into the stenosis and can potentially provide better results with dilatation before stenting (see later section). Lasers are also used for the debridement of obstructive lesions of recurrent respiratory papillomatosis and produces minimal scarring despite repetitive use. The CO_2 laser is also used as a treatment for glottic webs or for acquired subglottic stenosis.[21,25]

The neodymium:yttrium-aluminum-garnet (Nd:YAG) laser has become the laser of choice in the treatment of obstructing tracheal lesions because it is able to reach distant corners of the tracheobronchial anatomy. This laser can be used in concentric stenoses and in palliation of tracheal malignancies. However, endoscopists are unable to control the depth of penetration (up to 10 mm, depending on wattage and exposure time) with this type of laser, putting patients at risk for perforation.[25]

The potassium titanyl phosphate (KTP) or argon laser has also been used in the airway. The KTP laser is frequently used in the small pediatric airway because of its small diameter fibers and its coagulating effect on soft tissue.[23] It has a tissue penetration of 4 mm and is useful for vascular lesions as well. The KTP laser can be used with a fiberoptic delivery system, making its delivery more precise.[25] Lasers cannot destroy the root of the tumor, and recurrence is frequent after laser tumor ablation. If definitive surgical treatment is to be undertaken for patients, lasers should not be used because they can destroy healthy tissue that is adjacent to the lesion, which could compromise future anastomotic sites for the surgeon.[24]

Although not the focus of this article, it needs to be stressed that before any laser or cautery use in the airway, typical safety precautions need to occur. These include lowering the FiO_2 to below 30%, ensuring that the endotracheal tube (ETT) or other combustible materials are well away from the laser, and the universal donning of laser protective glasses.

Stents

Stents can have multiple uses in this patient population. They can be used as palliation for patients who have tumors that are too extensive for surgery, patients with benign lesions but extensive strictures, or patients with trachea destroyed by multiple reconstruction attempts. They can be used as temporizing measures until the patient is ready for surgery or as an adjunct to surgery to stabilize the newly anastomosed trachea.[24] Ideally, stents must have several characteristics: they should reestablish the airway with minimal morbidity and mortality, have limited migration, be easily removable, maintain luminal patency without ischemia or erosion, induce minimal granulation tissue formation, and be economically affordable.[26] But no stent currently satisfies all of these characteristics.

The advantage of an airway stent is that it supports the airway wall against collapse or external compression and impedes extension of tumor into the airway lumen. Stents can be safely used in patients undergoing external beam radiation therapy or brachytherapy; however, they can burn or break when subjected to Nd:YAG laser energy, the effects of electrocautery, or the effects of argon plasma coagulation.

Silicone stents, such as the Dumon (Endoxan prosthetics, Ayton, France) and Hood brands (Pembroke, MA, USA), protect from collapse and ingrowth of tumors.[26] Silicone is the least irritating of the stent materials, so there is less associated inflammation. Silicone stents are easily removed and exchanged, resist external compression, and cause minimal formation of granulation tissue. However, their more rigid structure cannot conform to irregular airways. The most common complication seen with silicone stent is migration of the stent, followed by granulation formation and mucous plugging. Other complications include malposition, infection, or obstruction related to inflammatory tissue overgrowth.[23]

Metal stents provide an advantage in that they are less likely to inhibit the respiratory cilia compared with silicone stents. In early generations, these metal stents required a balloon to expand after the stent was placed in the proper position. With the use of self-expanding stents, a balloon is no longer needed. Expandable stents are made of woven wire struts or meshes, typically from alloys such as nitinol. They can be positioned using bronchoscopy. However, tumor ingrowth can occur along the length of the stent. Also, these stents are extremely difficult to remove, may collapse or fracture with increased external pressure along the stent, and have ingrowth of granulation tissue that may lead to lumen occlusion.[26]

The covered self-expanding metallic stents are considered hybrids of metallic and silicone stents. They have a decreased risk for tumor ingrowth and granulation tissue because the wire mesh is covered with synthetic material. However, the ends are still uncovered to provide anchoring into the mucosa. As a result of their uncovered metal ends, these stents have less migration than their silicone counterparts. However, they also have an increased risk of granulation tissue formation at the ends compared with the silicone stents.[23,26] Because of the formation of granulation tissue, metallic stents are ideally used in cases of malignant strictures, and silicone stents are reserved for use in the treatment of benign strictures.

All stents can be inserted and removed endoscopically under general anesthesia or while awake and sedated with local anesthetic topicalization of the airway. Stents can be inserted using fluoroscopic guidance with bronchoscopic assistance. Broncho-scopic evaluation during stent placement allows insertion of a guidewire across the stricture. Bronchoscopy can again be used after stent placement to evaluate patency and location of the stent. If incorrectly positioned, the stent may be repositioned with bronchoscopy forceps.[26,27]

Anesthesia for stent placement

An experienced anesthesiology team working in close cooperation with the surgeon or interventional pulmonologist is required for optimal care. Sedative pre-medication should only be used for very anxious patients because of the danger of hypoventilation and further airway obstruction. An anticholinergic agent can be selected as part of the premedication to decrease excessive airway secretions.[28] It is important to remember that in changing a spontaneously breathing patient to positive pressure ventilation, a partially obstructing lesion can completely obstruct the airway. Also, the bronchoscope may completely obstruct the airway when entering the area of stenosis. Both of these issues make preoxygenation vital before starting the procedure. Because of altered airflow, preoxygenation/denitro-genation will take considerably longer than usual. Tidal breathing may be inhibited, and 5 maximal breaths in a patient with a compromised trachea will be insufficient for effective nitrogen washout.

Sedation can be provided without airway compromise, using agents such as dex-medetomidine or ketamine. Dexmedetomidine was initially described as a possible agent for sedation by Hall and colleagues.[29] They took 7 volunteers and found that hemodynamics, oxygen saturation, and respiratory rate were well preserved during the infusion of the drug, whereas most patients experienced amnesia and sedation. The use of dexmedetomidine for the management of difficult airways has been docu-mented with success in other case reports.[30,31] Candiotti and colleagues[32] describe the use of dexmedetomidine for monitored anesthesia care in a randomized, double-blind trial. This trial found that patients undergoing sedation with dexmedeto-midine required less fentanyl, had less respiratory depression, and had increased satisfaction with the anesthesia care. It is important to note that dexmedetomidine can result in significant bradycardia and hypotension.

For initial bronchoscopy, local anesthetics can be used to anesthetize the airway. Practitioners may have different ways of doing this. However, local anesthetics are not without their own consequences. They may decrease forced expiratory volume in the first second of expiration and forced vital capacity, further exacerbating the inspiratory airflow limitation by inhibiting airway dilator responses and may cause deep sedation when absorbed in significant quantity. One must also be cautious of total local anesthetics used because these are easily absorbed through mucosal membranes, and toxic levels can be reached.[33,34] Airflow limitation secondary to local anesthesia of the airway may lead to complete airway obstruction in a compromised airway.

In a patient with significant stenosis who presents with respiratory compromise, the logical first step is to dilate the stricture under minimal anesthetic. Even though the dilatation will not last, this initial step will produce a patient in whom the airway is not critically narrowed so that other diagnostic tests and preoperative preparation can take place. Further, linear cautery of the stenosis and balloon dilatation may produce less inflammation and edema as compared with extensive laser therapy; so the patient would have less risk of acute airway compromise.[26,35]

Induction of anesthesia needs to be tailored to the patients' lesions and their medical history. Traditionally, it is recommended to avoid neuromuscular blockade and maintain a patient ventilating spontaneously. However, others state that control of the airway is best after an intravenous induction with an agent such as propofol and a short acting neuromuscular blocker.[35] The extent and the fixed versus dynamic characteristics of the stenosis can help guide anesthetic choices. Periglottic dynamic collapse can potentially make intubation difficult, and thus, maintenance of muscular tone and spontaneous respiration may be advantageous. Similarly, immediate subglottic stenoses can make seating of an ETT impossible. In these cases, awake sedated bronchoscopy leading to control of the airway is recommended. Laryngeal mask airways (LMAs) can be placed in patients with proximal lesions to allow ventilation/oxygenation and access for fiberoptic bronchoscopy.

If intravenous induction is chosen, the medications are tailored to the patient's health, the type and duration of the surgery, and the type of airway therapy used. Regimens are typical for all critically ill patients. Total intravenous anesthesia (TIVA) with propofol and remifentanil is useful when rigid bronchoscopy is expected (these should be rapidly available in any case). Obtundation of airway reflexes with opioids needs to be balanced against potential CO_2 retention in patients with COPD. Typical doses of 2 to 4 mg/kg fentanyl help to maintain hemodynamic stability throughout the procedure. Titrated doses of propofol, ketamine, or etomidate can then be added. The focus of induction is shifted toward rapid controlling of the airway, because mask ventilation may be difficult with the higher required pressures causing gastric distension. If mask ventilation is attempted or necessary,a slower rate with longer inspiratory and expiratory times is required to allow for adequate tidal exchange.

For midtracheal stenoses, there is often room to seat an ETT cephalad to the stricture. Jet ventilation, either supraglottic or intraglottic, is an option. However, because of its nature, it is hard to raise the concentration of inspired oxygen, and the narrow orifice of the stenosis can dramatically inhibit the flow.

After the induction of anesthesia, passage of an ETT down the airway can be guided by a fiberoptic bronchoscope. An LMA can be placed to facilitate oxygenation/ventilation and bronchoscopic evaluation/treatment of proximal lesions. Regardless of the mode of induction chosen for the patient, an interventional pulmonologist or surgeon who is familiar with a rigid bronchoscope must always be ready to control the airway. In extreme cases of airway obstruction, percutaneous cardiopulmonary bypass may be instituted if airway control cannot be established with a rigid bronchoscope. Anesthesia for stent cases can be maintained using inhalational agent but is more commonly maintained using total intravenous anesthesia and short-acting agents such as remifentanil and propofol.[5,36] Intravenous agents maintain the depth of anesthesia during the frequent periods of suctioning, airway dilatation, and stenting when ventilation is interrupted. Patients may be ventilated with positive pressure ventilation of various modes that include common tidal volume or pressure control, jet ventilation, and high-frequency ventilation. Regardless of the type of anesthetic used during a case, a patient must be fully awake with intact airway reflexes at the end of the procedure.

Ventilation

As mentioned earlier, understanding the location and type of lesion will guide ventilatory management. Typical midtracheal stenotic lesions from ETT damage will require a decrease in respiratory rate to allow an increase in inspiratory and exhalation times. With higher inspiratory pressures made possible by intubation, it is reasonable that only the exhalation times would need to be lengthened because exhalation is a purely passive process. If hypotension is encountered after the initiation of positive pressure ventilation, differential diagnosis needs to include breath stacking due to obstructed exhalation, along with the more common issues of pneumothorax, drug effect, myocardial ischemia, and so on.

Jet ventilation is often used for diagnostic and therapeutic procedures. If the jet catheter is supraglottic, care must be taken to aim the jet at the lumen of the stenosis to avoid direct trauma to adjacent tissue. If the catheter is passed through the stenotic orifice, hyperinflation must be considered a constant threat. Prolonged jet ventilation will necessitate arterial CO_2 sampling along with standard monitoring.

The Montgomery T tube

The use of the T tube to treat tracheal stenosis was first reported by Dr Montgomery in 1964. Although considered a silicone stent, the Montgomery T tube is a specific device in that it serves both as a tracheal stent and a tracheostomy tube. The proximal (vertical) portion of the T tube extends above the tracheotomy, ending below the vocal cords in the region of the subglottic strictures. The distal (vertical) limb occupies the lumen of the upper and middle third of the trachea beneath the tracheotomy. The external (horizontal) limb protrudes through the tracheotomy site and serves as a portal for achieving pulmonary toilet and as a means of maintaining access to the trachea in case a tracheostomy tube needs to be placed for ventilatory support.[23,37] The T tube can be used in benign and malignant airway diseases and may be custom-tailored to stent across a stricture either via its proximal or distal limb. Like other airway stents, it may play a role as a bridge to definitive reconstruction, as an adjunct to primary surgical repair, or as definitive treatment in patients who cannot undergo surgical repair. Several techniques have been described for the placement of a T tube. Montgomery's original technique involves grasping the distal portion and advancing it to the distal trachea, doing the same with proximal end, and then pulling the extraluminal limb anteriorly. Other techniques were developed because this original technique could be technically challenging. The extraluminal limb can be plugged to preserve phonation and prevent dryness of respiratory mucosa.

Patients with T tubes may need general anesthesia for the assessment of tracheal lesions. This may be challenging for the anesthesia practitioner because ventilatory volume may escape the proximal end, risking hypoventilation, and there is no clear adapter for the extraluminal limb. To overcome the lack of proximal seal, a throat pack can be placed to limit volume loss through the proximal end, and the adapter to a 7 mm ETT can be put into the extraluminal (horizontal) limb. To access the proximal limb, an LMA can be placed. This allows a bronchoscope to be inserted via the LMA or the extraluminal limb. Both TIVA and inhalational anesthesia can be used.

SURGICAL MANAGEMENT
Tracheal Reconstruction

Resection and reconstruction with primary anastomosis may be undertaken in patients who fail dilatation and stent therapy. It is recommended that patients have a functional glottis and that those with neuromuscular disorders or profound pulmonary pathology be optimized so as to not require postoperative ventilation. Patients should not harbor active infection or be on steroids because these can lead to wound dehiscence. In tracheal resections, patients are usually positioned supine with the head of the bed elevated and the neck extended. A low-collar incision is made, and the pretracheal plane is entered and developed by blunt dissection. Distal tracheal lesions may require a partial sternotomy and/or right posterolateral thoracotomy for extended mobilization of the trachea and tracheal release maneuvers. These include the suprathyroid laryngeal release, suprahyoid laryngeal release, and right pulmonary hilar release.

The trachea is freed around its circumference only in the area of the stenosis; this prevents devascularization of the tracheal ends used for anastomosis. The trachea is entered below the area of stenosis and transected. At this time, the patient is ventilated by the intubation of the distal trachea across the operative field. Occasionally, it may be necessary for the patient to undergo brief periods of apnea for the surgeons to work. Alternatively, a jet catheter can be passed either through the endotracheal tube or across the field and into the distal trachea. TIVA is typically used during the resection. The surgical technique used must be tailored to the type and site of the stenosis. The surgeon then forms the anastomosis between the 2 free ends of the trachea. This anastomosis is tested for air leaks by submerging it under saline while pressurizing the airway to 25 to 40 cm of water. Either the air leaks are directly repaired or the anastomosis is restructured. A formal tracheostomy or a "Mini-Trach" for secretion management can be placed after closure. A chin-to-chest stitch may be placed to prevent hyperextension and excessive tension on the fresh anastomosis.[38]

Attempts should be made to extubate the patient in the operating room to prevent the fresh anastomosis from being exposed to high airway pressures. In the immediate postoperative procedure, patients may require flexible bronchoscopy to clear secretions or for the examination of the anastomosis. Edema is prevented by limiting the intake of fluids. In some cases of edema, patients may require steroids or reduced-density helium-oxygen mixtures.[5,38] Nebulized racemic epinephrine can also be useful to reduce airway swelling.

Anesthesia for tracheal resection

Much like the anesthesia for placements of stents, anesthesia for tracheal reconstruction surgery requires planning and good communication between the surgeon and the anesthesiologist because they must share control of the airway. A detailed preoperative history should include progression of the disease, history of prior intubations, and any other pertinent symptoms that the patient has experienced. Standard monitors of electrocardiogram, oxygen saturation, blood pressure, and capnography should be used. It is recommended to place an arterial line in the left arm in these patients because their innominate artery may be operatively manipulated or compressed, thus making pressure readings in the right arm inaccurate. The premedication and induction of anesthesia should be approached in the same way as that for pulmonary stent placements. Although no adverse effects were seen with an intravenous induction using neuromuscular blocker, others prefer to maintain a patient ventilating spontaneously until the airway is secured.

Besides induction, the other challenge that the anesthesiology team encounters is how to ventilate an open airway. As described by Pinsonneault and colleagues,[24] 5 different modes of ventilation can be used during these procedures. Manual oxygen jet ventilation or low-frequency jet ventilation requires the anesthesiologist to manually trigger O_2 delivery under high pressure. This form of ventilation allows free access to the surgical field, but it can lead to hypercarbia due to hypoventilation. The lungs can also be ventilated using high-frequency ventilation: high-frequency positive pressure ventilation, high-frequency jet ventilation, or high-frequency oscillation ventilation. High-frequency positive pressure ventilation delivers very small tidal volumes using a ventilator at 1 breath per minute. With high-frequency jet ventilation, pulses of gas at 50 psi are delivered. Air entrainment occurs with high-frequency jet ventilation, leading to a lower concentration of oxygen delivery. High-frequency ventilation results in good gas exchange, decreases the risk of atelectasis secondary to auto–positive end-expiratory pressure, and results in minimal hemodynamic changes. The surgeon also has an unobstructed field with this type of ventilation. No single form of ventilation is preferred, but it is important to discuss and plan how to proceed with ventilating the open airway with the surgeon before the induction of anesthesia.

CASE DISCUSSION

MS was a 57-year-old man who was admitted with increasing shortness of breath and a tracheal stricture found on bronchoscopy by a referring pulmonologist. He had a medical history of hypertension, hypercholesterolemia, coronary artery disease, and peripheral vascular disease with claudication. Two weeks before admission, he underwent peripheral vascular surgery at an outside institution. He had multiple intubation attempts. His postoperative course was benign. He was repeatedly treated for reactive airways disease during his 3-day hospitalization. His shortness of breath rapidly progressed during the ensuing week.

MS presented with complaints or dyspnea. He had audible wheezing on inspiration and exhalation. He appeared to be working hard on inspiration and exhalation. He was receiving nasal cannula oxygen at 6 L/min, with an oxygen saturation of 92%. With a known diagnosis of tracheal stenosis, his therapy was changed to helium 75%/oxygen 25%. Although his arterial oxygen saturation did not change, his work of breathing and his complaints of dyspnea decreased. Physical examination at this time revealed mild inspiratory and expiratory stridor greatest over the sternal notch and transmitted to the distal airways. It increased greatly in volume when the patient was taken off the oxygen and placed on nasal cannula. A CT scan with 3D reconstruction (**Figs. 2** and **3**) indicated a narrowing and an anterior shift of narrowed segment. Such a shift in the airway configuration as a result of the fibrosis can cause turbulent airflow and increased work of breathing even in the absence of narrowing. Further, such a change in the axis of the airway can make airway control more difficult because the endotracheal tube may not be able to follow the serpentine airway.

MS was brought to the operating room for initial evaluation with awake flexible fiberoptic bronchoscopy and dilatation. His nasal and oral airways were topicalized in standard fashion. **Fig. 4** is the preinterventional bronchoscopy; this shows 2 areas of narrowing and the nonlinear nature of the trachea. An initial management plan of serial dilatations with rigid bronchoscopy for several weeks was planned with close follow-up to determine if stenosis recurred and resection was needed. For this procedure, the patient was induced and an LMA placed. An LMA was chosen because the authors were uncertain if there was sufficient room for the endotracheal tip and cuff between the vocal cords and the stenosis. Neuromuscular blockade was chosen to allow

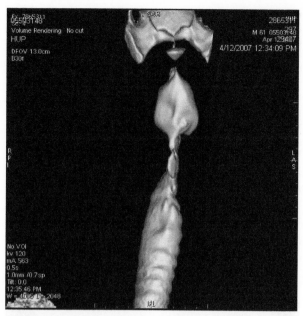

Fig. 2. A 3D reconstructed axial image of a patient with subglottic tracheal stenosis.

a slow respiratory rate (prolonged inspiratory and exhalation time), without the hypotension associated with the depth of anesthesia necessary for lack of spontaneous ventilation. Further, the authors desired paralysis so that there would be no risk of negative pressure pulmonary edema when the airway was obstructed with the dilating

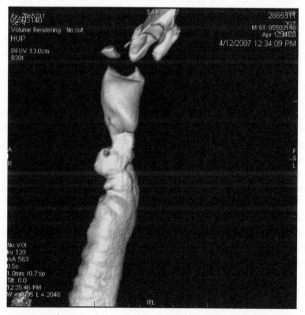

Fig. 3. A 3D reconstructed sagittal image of a patient with subglottic tracheal stenosis.

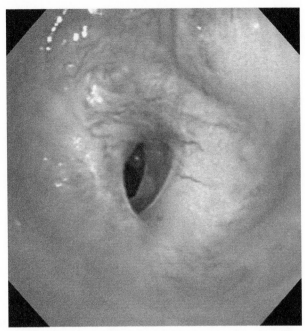

Fig. 4. Bronchoscopic view of tracheal stenosis seen in **Figs. 2** and **3**. The location of the stenosis and its smooth and circumferential presentation suggest an injury from a tracheal balloon.

balloon. The operating room was set up for immediate rigid bronchoscopy should airway compromise occur. The patient received intravenous steroids to prevent or minimize airway edema.

The patient was maintained on 30% oxygen for airway cautery. The stenotic area was incised in 4 places with cautery (3, 6, 9, and 12 o'clock). The patient was then switched to 100% oxygen in preparation for dilatation. Three serial dilatations with a saline-filled balloon resulted in dramatically improved ventilation. The patient was then switched to TIVA for rigid bronchoscopy. Serial dilatation with 5 mm, 6 mm, and 7 mm (internal diameter) rigid bronchoscopes was undertaken. Ventilation occurred by coaxial jet ventilation. After hemostasis was achieved and the airway was suctioned, the rigid scope was removed and an LMA was placed for final flexible bronchoscopy and termination of anesthesia.

In the recovery room, the patient was immediately treated with racemic epinephrine. He was discharged home on a 5-day Solu-Medrol dose pack. The patient remained well and 1 week later returned for a repeat bronchoscopy (**Fig. 5**). The patient was dilated again. But the patient's symptoms and stenosis recurred, although much less than initial presentation, and a definitive tracheal resection was planned.

For the formal tracheal resection, general anesthesia was induced and an LMA was placed. The surgeons repeatedly measured the distance from the carina to the distal end of the stenosis, the length of the stenosis, and the distance from the proximal end of the stenosis to the vocal cords. This enabled the surgeons to determine how many tracheal rings would be resected and the type, if any, of tracheal release that would be done. An arterial line was placed and the trachea was intubated with a 5-mm ETT. The arms were tucked and padded.

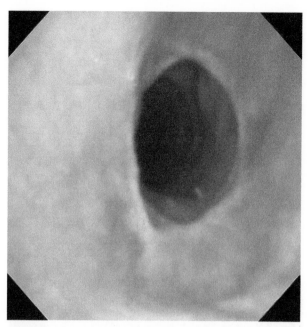

Fig. 5. The stenosis from **Fig. 4** 1 week after endobronchial therapy. The invasive pulmonologists had made a series of radial cuts into the stenosis to control the tearing when they balloon dilated.

After the trachea was exposed, the bronchoscope was placed into the ETT and slowly withdrawn to the proximal stenosis. Under bronchoscopic view, a needle was placed into the trachea to give an external landmark for the distal end of the stenosis. The distal trachea was divided and TIVA was started. Ventilation was by a 6-mm anode ETT, and a sterile ventilator circuit passed off the field. The transoral 5-mm ETT was retracted and left in place below the vocal cords. Once the stenotic lesion was excised, a jet ventilation catheter was placed through the transoral ETT and into the distal trachea. The narrow diameter of the catheter allowed the surgeon the access to the posterior wall of the trachea for reconstruction. During this portion, the authors were concerned for any arrhythmias as a result of rising arterial CO_2 concentration. If this were to occur, the transoral ETT would have been guided into the distal trachea by the surgeon for tidal ventilation, whereas other causes of instability were ruled out.

Once the posterior wall of the trachea was reapproximated, the transoral ETT was advanced across the suture line until the balloon was distal to the suture line. Tidal ventilation was resumed, and the trachea and neck were closed. Because the trachea was shortened by 2 rings, the patient's neck was flexed to remove tension. A stitch was placed from the patient's chin to the chest to guard the patient against extending their head. The ETT was removed, and the LMA was placed instead. Bronchoscopy showed a widely open tracheal lumen (**Fig. 6**). However, if at this point there was a question about the repair or a concern about the patient's ability to cough and control airway secretions, a tracheostomy or a minitracheostomy would have been placed.

The back of the operating room table was raised and pillows were used to reinforce the neck's flexed position. Spontaneous ventilation was allowed, and the LMA was

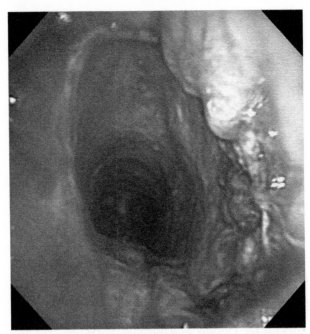

Fig. 6. Because the therapy from **Fig. 5** was temporary and the patient suffered a recurrence of stenosis, they had tracheal surgery with resection of 2 tracheal rings and primary reanastomosis. The carina is visible in the distance. There is some granulation tissue along the right suture margin that did not progress to requiring therapy.

removed. Once in the recovery room, the patient received a nebulized racemic epinephrine treatment. The patient was transferred to a high-acuity floor with respiratory rate checks every 15 minutes overnight.

SUMMARY

Tracheal stenosis may occur secondary to trauma, tumors, infection, inflammatory diseases, or iatrogenic causes. Understanding these lesions requires a basic understanding of the physics of airflow. All of these patients must be carefully evaluated and require a series of tests, including pulmonary function tests and radiographic studies. Treatment of tracheal lesions is a multidisciplinary issue and requires the close participation of interventional pulmonologists, anesthesiologists, and surgeons.

REFERENCES

1. Lorenz RR, Netterville JL, Burkey BB. Head and neck. In: Townsend CB, Beauchamp RD, Evers BM, et al, editors. Sabiston textbook of surgery: the biological basis of modern surgical practice. 18th edition. Philadelphia: Saunders Elsevier; 2008.
2. Cantrell JR, Guild HG. Congenital stenosis of the trachea. Am J Surg 1964;108: 297–305.
3. Gamsu G, Borson DB, Webb WR, et al. Structure and function in tracheal stenosis. Am Rev Respir Dis 1980;121:519–31.

4. Grenier PA, Beigelman-Aubry C, Brillet PY, et al. Nonneoplastic tracheal and bronchial stenoses. Radiol Clin North Am 2009;47:243–60.
5. Ashiku SK, Mathisen DJ. Idiopathic laryngotracheal stenosis. Chest Surg Clin N Am 2003;13:257–69.
6. Hagberg C, Georgi R, Krier C, et al. Complications of managing the airway. Best Pract Res Clin Anaesthesiol 2005;19:641–59.
7. Spittle N, McCluskey A. Lesson of the week: tracheal stenosis after intubation [comment]. BMJ 2000;321:1000–2.
8. Cooper JD, Grillo HC. The evolution of tracheal injury due to ventilatory assistance through cuffed tubes: a pathologic study. Ann Surg 1969;169: 334–48.
9. Cooper JD, Grillo HC. Experimental production and prevention of injury due to cuffed tracheal tubes. Surg Gynecol Obstet 1969;129:1235–41.
10. Stauffer JL, Olson DE, Petty TL, et al. Complications and consequences of endotracheal intubation and tracheotomy. A prospective study of 150 critically ill adult patients. Am J Med 1981;70:65–76.
11. Bogdasarian RS, Olson NR. Posterior glottic laryngeal stenosis. Otolaryngol Head Neck Surg 1980;88(6):765–72.
12. Kandaswamy C, Balasubramanian V. Review of adult tracheomalacia and its relationship with chronic obstructive pulmonary disease. Curr Opin Pulm Med 2009; 15:113–9.
13. Cansiz H, Yener M, Tahamiler R, et al. Preoperative detection and management of tracheomalacia in advanced laryngotracheal stenosis. B-ENT 2008;4:163–7.
14. Hess DR, Fink JB, Venkataraman ST, et al. The history and physics of heliox. Respir Care 2006;51:608–12.
15. Wain JC. Postintubation tracheal stenosis. Chest Surg Clin N Am 2003;13: 231–46.
16. Dueck R. Assessment and monitoring of flow limitation and other parameters from flow/volume loops. J Clin Monit Comput 2000;16:425–32.
17. Culver BH. Pulmonary function and exercise testing. In: Albert RK, Spiro SG, Jett JR, editors. Clinical respiratory medicine. 2nd edition. Philadelphia: Elsevier Saunders; 2004. p. 117–28.
18. Lunn WW, Sheller JR. Flow volume loops in the evaluation of upper airway obstruction. Otolaryngol Clin North Am 1995;28:721–9.
19. Kryger M, Bode F, Antic R, et al. Diagnosis of obstruction of the upper and central airways. Am J Med 1976;61:85–93.
20. Feller-Kopman D. Acute complications of artificial airways. Clin Chest Med 2003; 24:445–55.
21. Bolliger CT, Sutedja TG, Strausz J, et al. Therapeutic bronchoscopy with immediate effect: laser, electrocautery, argon plasma coagulation and stents [comment]. Eur Respir J 2006;27:1258–71.
22. Prince JS, Duhamel DR, Levin DL, et al. Nonneoplastic lesions of the tracheobronchial wall: radiologic findings with bronchoscopic correlation. [Erratum appears in Radiographics 2003;23(1):191]. Radiographics 2002;22(Spec No): S215–30.
23. Shapshay SM, Valdez TA. Bronchoscopic management of benign stenosis. Chest Surg Clin N Am 2001;11:749–68.
24. Pinsonneault C, Fortier J, Donati F, et al. Tracheal resection and reconstruction. Can J Anaesth 1999;46:439–55.
25. Lando T, April MM, Ward RF, et al. Minimally invasive techniques in laryngotracheal reconstruction. Otolaryngol Clin North Am 2008;41:935–46.

26. Chin CS, Litle V, Yun J, et al. Airway stents. Ann Thorac Surg 2008;85:S792–6.
27. Shin JH, Song HY, Shim TS, et al. Management of tracheobronchial strictures. Cardiovasc Intervent Radiol 2004;27:314–24.
28. Brodsky JB. Anesthesia for pulmonary stent insertion. Curr Opin Anaesthesiol 2003;16:3.
29. Hall JE, Uhrich TD, Barney JA, et al. Sedative, amnestic, and analgesic properties of small-dose dexmedetomidine infusions. Anesth Analg 2000;90:699–705.
30. Bergese SD, Khabiri B, Roberts WD, et al. Dexmedetomidine for conscious sedation in difficult awake fiberoptic intubation cases [comment]. [Erratum appears in J Clin Anesth 2007;19(4):323]. J Clin Anesth 2007;19:141–4.
31. Grant SA, Breslin DS, MacLeod DB, et al. Dexmedetomidine infusion for sedation during fiberoptic intubation: a report of three cases. J Clin Anesth 2004;16:124–6.
32. Candiotti KA, Bergese SD, Bokesch PM, et al. Monitored anesthesia care with dexmedetomidine: a prospective, randomized, double-blind, multicenter trial. Anesth Analg 2010;110(1):47–56.
33. Ho AM, Chung DC, Karmakar MK, et al. Dynamic airflow limitation after topical anaesthesia of the upper airway. Anaesth Intensive Care 2006;34:211–5.
34. Kuna ST, Woodson GE, Sant'Ambrogio G, et al. Effect of laryngeal anesthesia on pulmonary function testing in normal subjects. Am Rev Respir Dis 1988;137:656–61.
35. Conacher ID. Anaesthesia and tracheobronchial stenting for central airway obstruction in adults [comment]. Br J Anaesth 2003;90:367–74.
36. Finlayson GN, Brodsky JB. Anesthetic considerations for airway stenting in adult patients. Anesthesiol Clin 2008;26:281–91.
37. Wahidi MM, Ernst A. The Montgomery T-tube tracheal stent. Clin Chest Med 2003;24:437–43.
38. Lorenz RR. Adult laryngotracheal stenosis: etiology and surgical management. Curr Opin Otolaryngol Head Neck Surg 2003;11:467–72.

Index

Note: Page numbers of article titles are in **boldface** type.

Anesthesiology Clin 28 (2010) 175–183
doi:10.1016/S1932-2275(10)00035-2   **anesthesiology.theclinics.com**
1932-2275/10/$ – see front matter © 2010 Elsevier Inc. All rights reserved.

Printed and bound by CPI Group (UK) Ltd, Croydon, CR0 4YY

03/10/2024

01040441-0018